Plant-Based Desserts on a Budget

Cheap and Tasty Desserts Recipes to Boost Your Diet and Manage Your Weight

I0145953

Clay Palmer

professional before attempting any techniques outlined in this book.

By reading this document, the reader agrees that under no circumstances is the author responsible for any losses, direct or indirect, which are incurred as a result of the use of information contained within this document, including, but not limited to, — errors, omissions, or inaccuracies.

Table of Contents

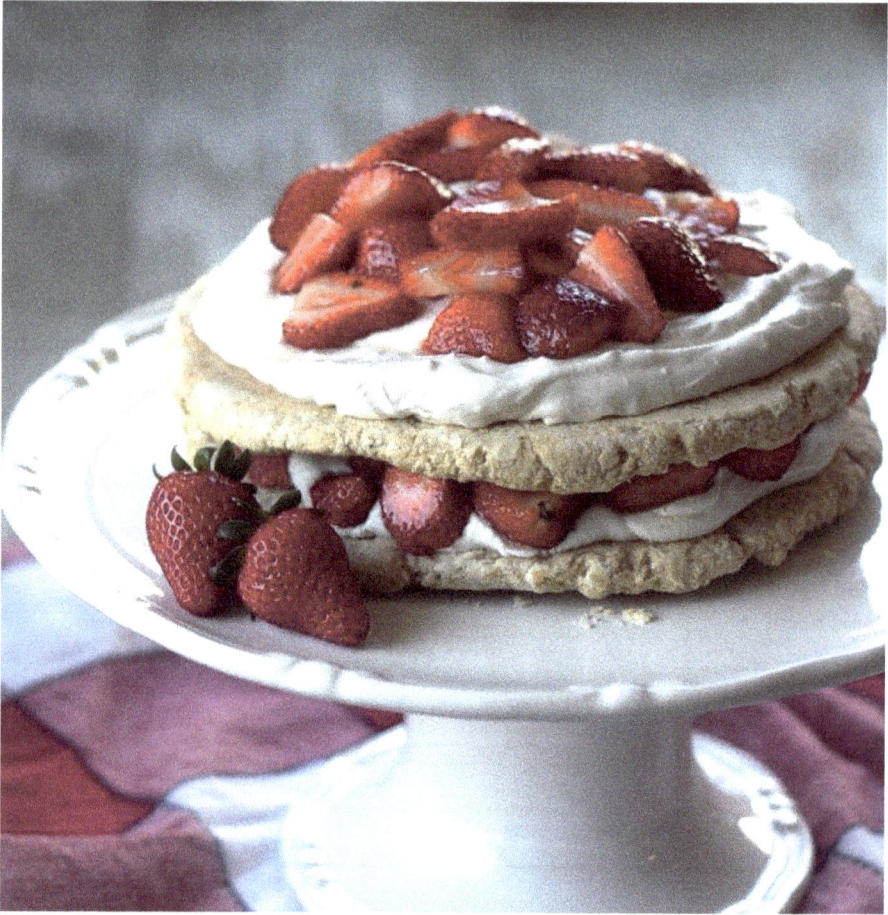

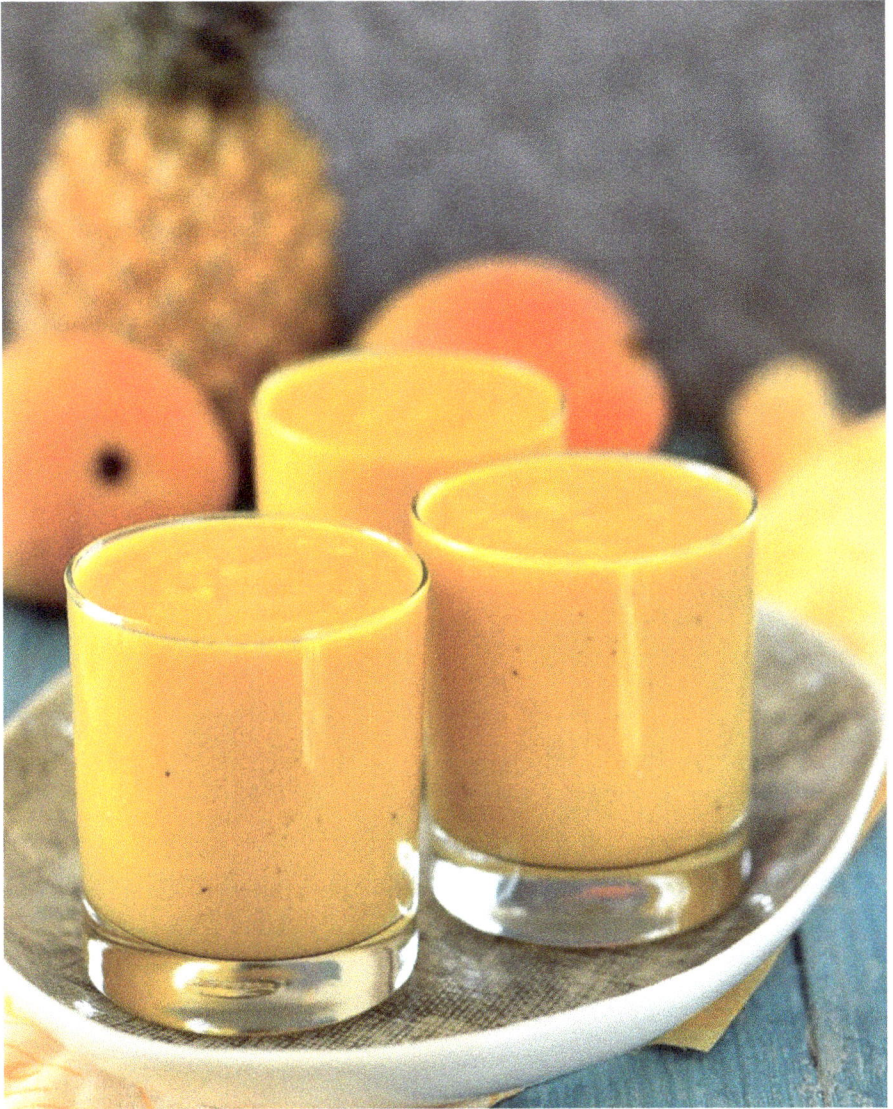

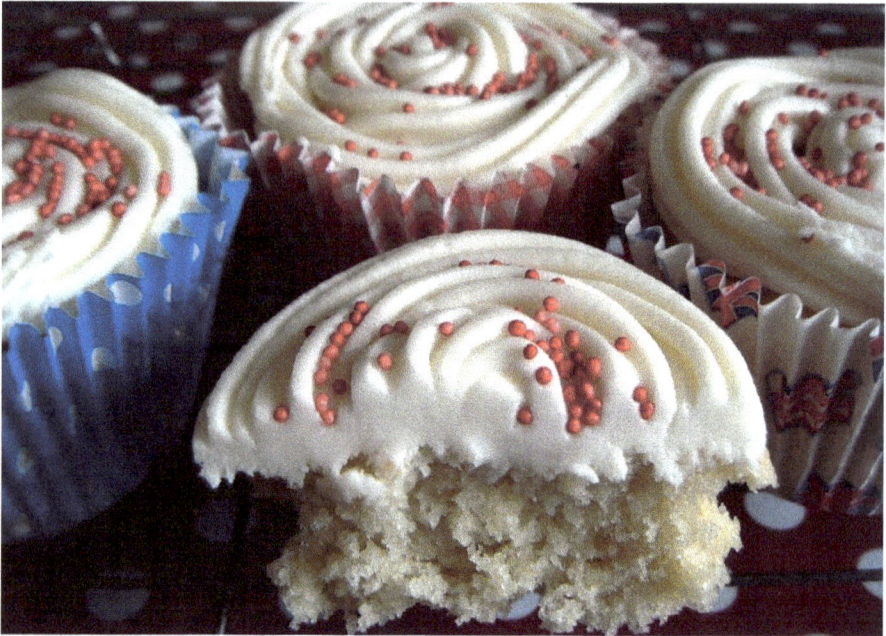

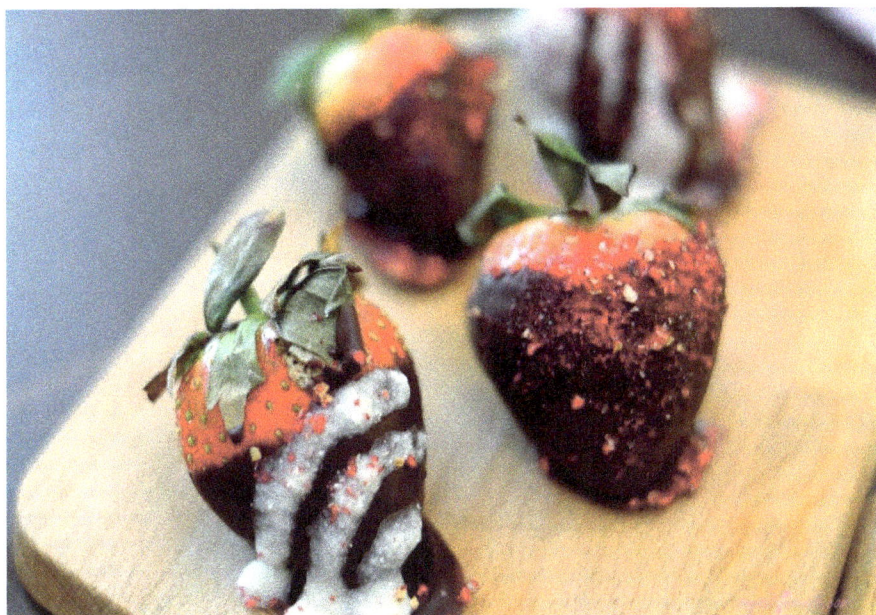

Raspberry-Flavored Chai Smoothie

Preparation time: 5 minutes Cooking time: 0 minutes Servings: 1

Ingredients:

1 black tea bag ¼ tsp ginger ¼ tsp cardamom powder ¼ cup coconut milk 2 tbsps raspberries What you'll need from the store cupboard: 2 packets Stevia or as desired 1 ¼ cups boiling water ¼ tsp cinnamon 3 tbsps MCT oil or coconut oil

Directions Add all ingredients in a blender. Blend until smooth and creamy. Serve and enjoy.

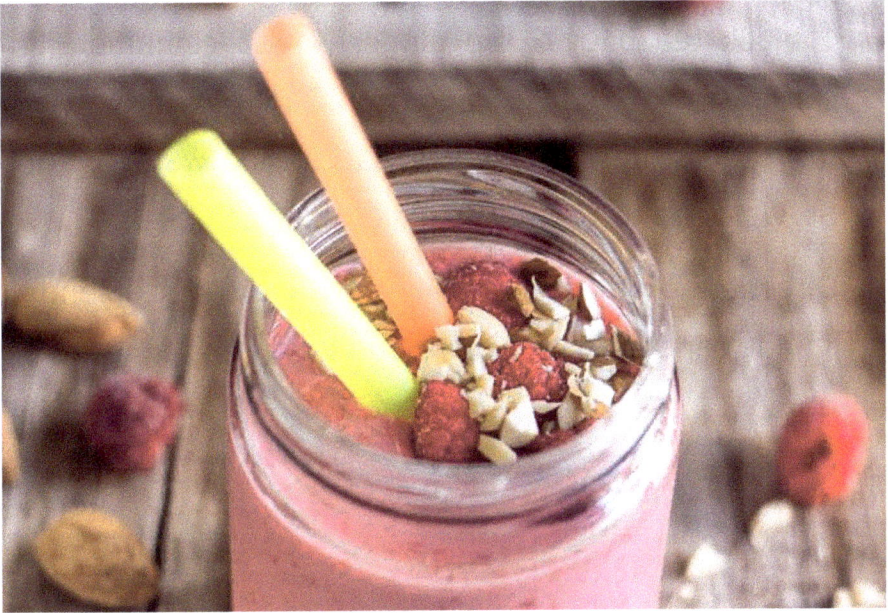

Chai Tea Smoothie

Preparation time: 5 minutes Cooking time: 0 minutes Servings: 1

Ingredients:

1 black tea bag ¼ tsp ginger ¼ tsp cinnamon ¼ tsp cardamom powder ½ cup coconut milk What you'll need from the store cupboard: 1 cup boiling water 2 packets Stevia or as desired 3 tbsp MCT oil or coconut oil

Directions Add all ingredients in a blender. Blend until smooth and creamy. Serve and enjoy.

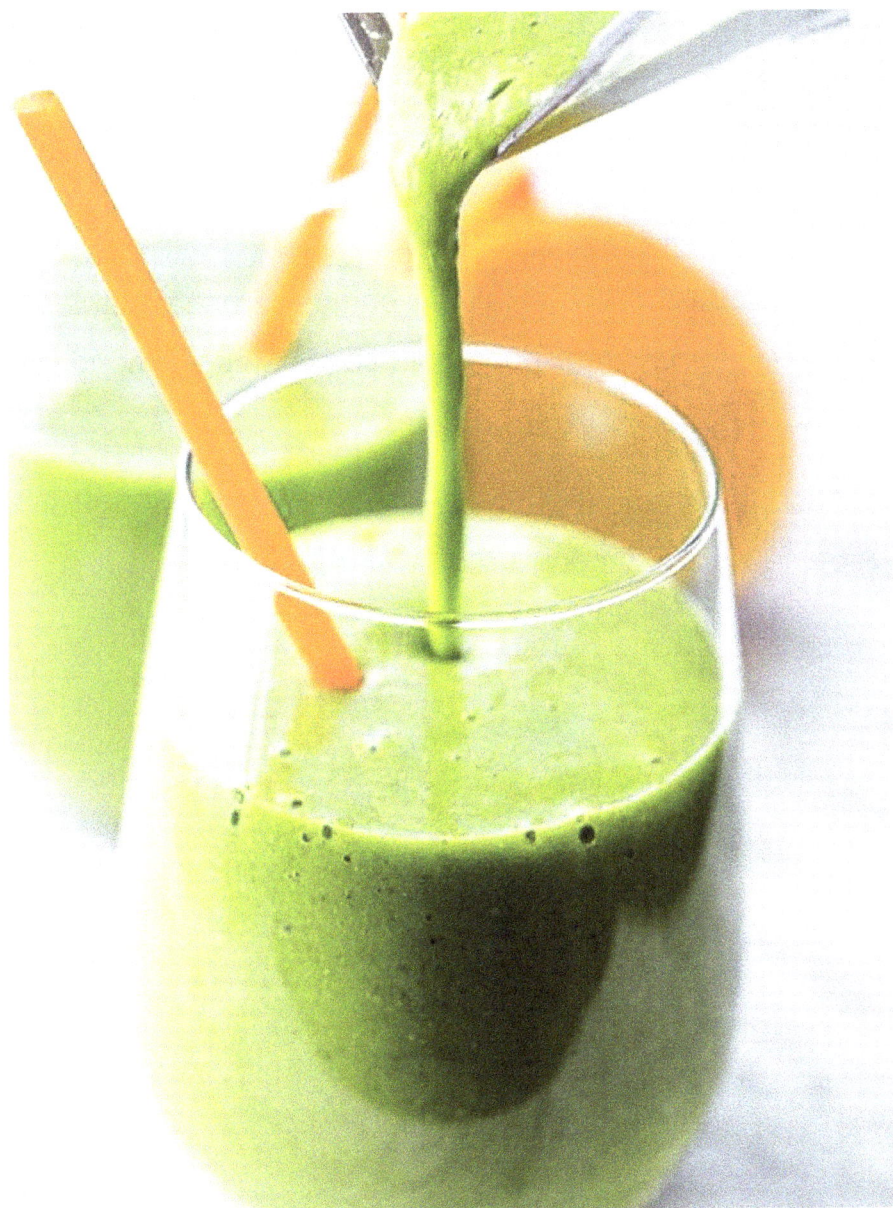

Hemp Green Smoothie

Preparation time: 30 minutes Cooking time: 0 minutes Servings: 01

Ingredients:

½ cup spinach ¼ avocado ½ banana, frozen 1 tablespoon hemp hearts 1 teaspoon chia seeds 1 cup almond milk

Directions:

Add all ingredients to a blender. Hit the pulse button and blend till it is smooth. Chill well to serve.

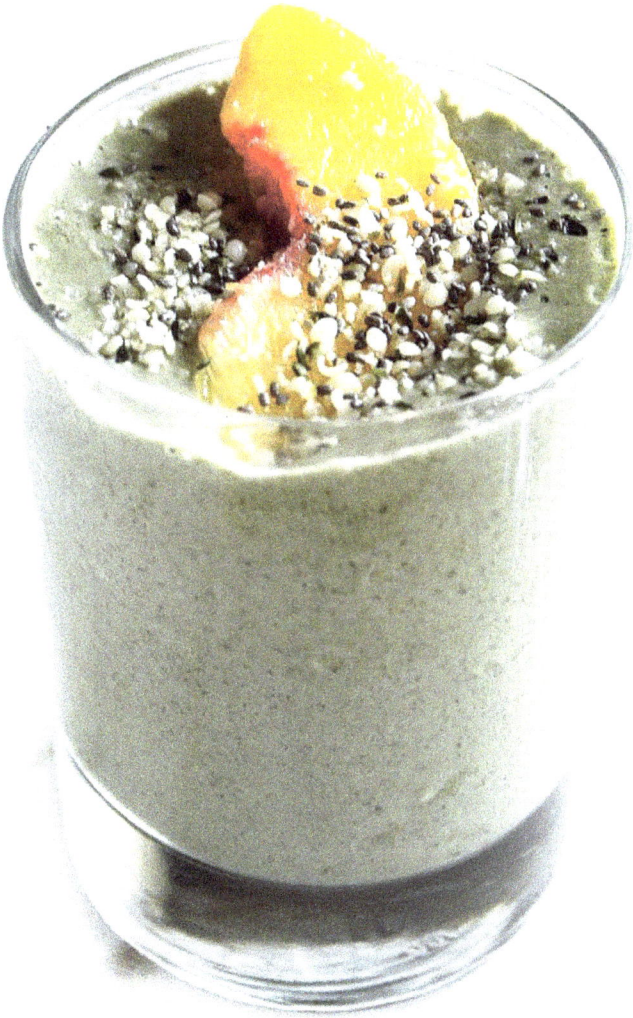

Gritty Choco Milk Shake

Preparation time:

5 minutes Cooking time: 0 minutes Servings: 1

Ingredients:

¼ cup heavy cream 1 tbsp chia seeds 1 tbsp hemp seeds 1 tbsp flaxseed 1 tbsp flaxseed oil What you'll need from the store cupboard: 1 ½ cups water 1 packet Stevia, or more to taste 1 tbsp cocoa powder 3 tbsp coconut oil

Directions

Add all ingredients in a blender. Blend until smooth and creamy. Serve and enjoy.

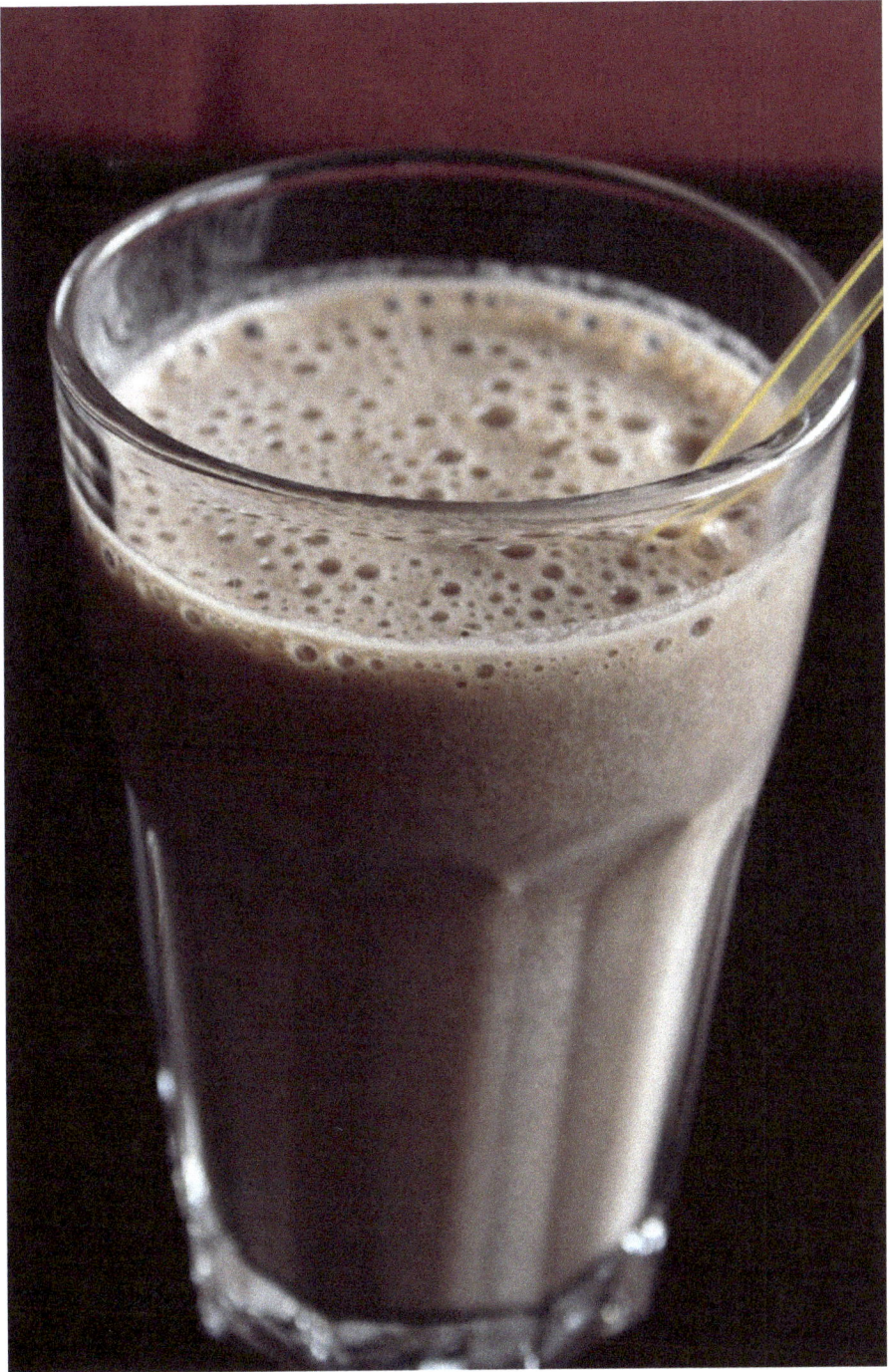

High Protein, Green and Fruity Smoothie

Preparation time: 10 minutes Cooking time: 0 minutes Servings: 2

Ingredients:

1 cup spinach, packed ½ small banana, peeled and frozen ½ avocado, peeled, pitted, and frozen 1 tbsp almond butter ¼ cup packed kale, stem discarded, and leaves chopped What you'll need from the store cupboard: 1 cup ice-cold water 5 tablespoons MCT oil or coconut oil

Directions

Whisk all ingredients in a blender until smooth and creamy. Serve and enjoy.

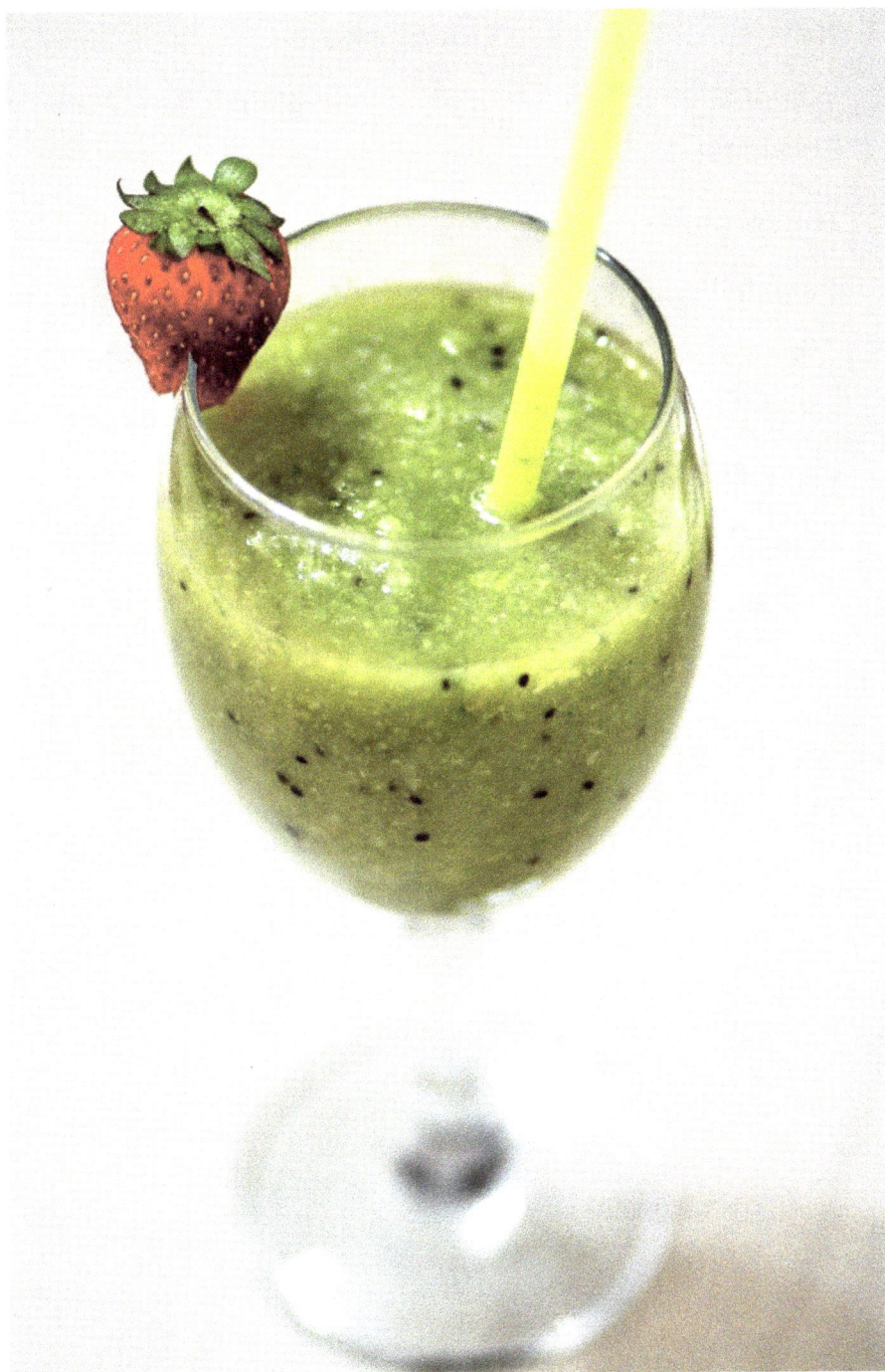

Nutritiously Green Milk Shake

Preparation time: 10 minutesCooking time: 5 minutes Servings: 1

Ingredients:

1 cup coconut cream 1 packet Stevia, or more to taste 1 tbsp coconut flakes, unsweetened 2 cups spring mix salad 3 tbsps coconut oil What you'll need from the store cupboard: 1 cup water

Directions Add all ingredients in a mixer. Whisk until smooth and creamy. Serve and enjoy.

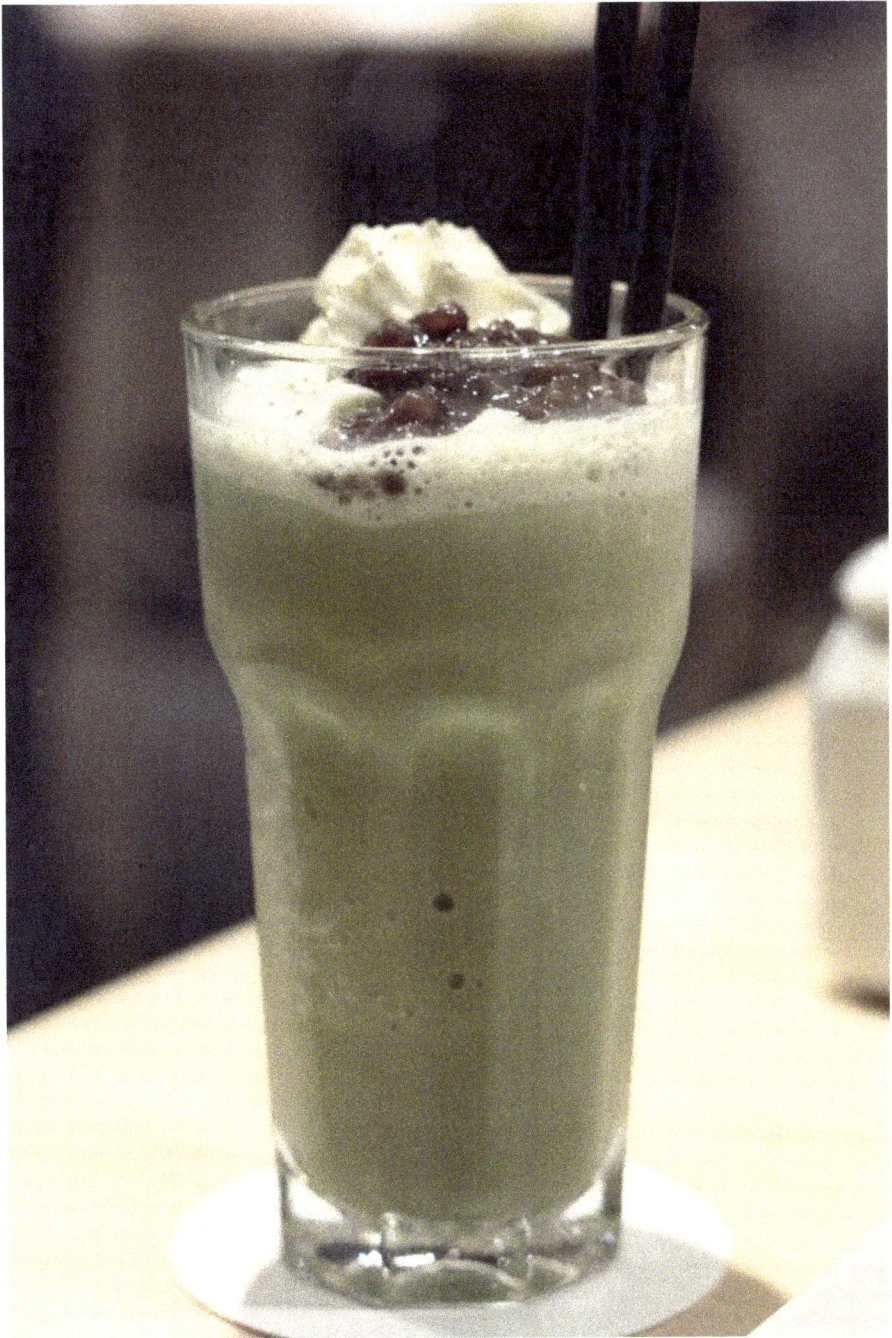

Raspberry and Greens Shake

Preparation time: 5 minutesCooking time: 0 minutes

Servings: 1

Ingredients:

½ cup half and half 1 packet Stevia, or more to taste 4 raspberries, fresh 1 tbsp macadamia oil 1 cup Spinach What you'll need from the store cupboard: 1 cup water

Directions

Add all ingredients in a mixer. Whisk until smooth and creamy. Serve and enjoy

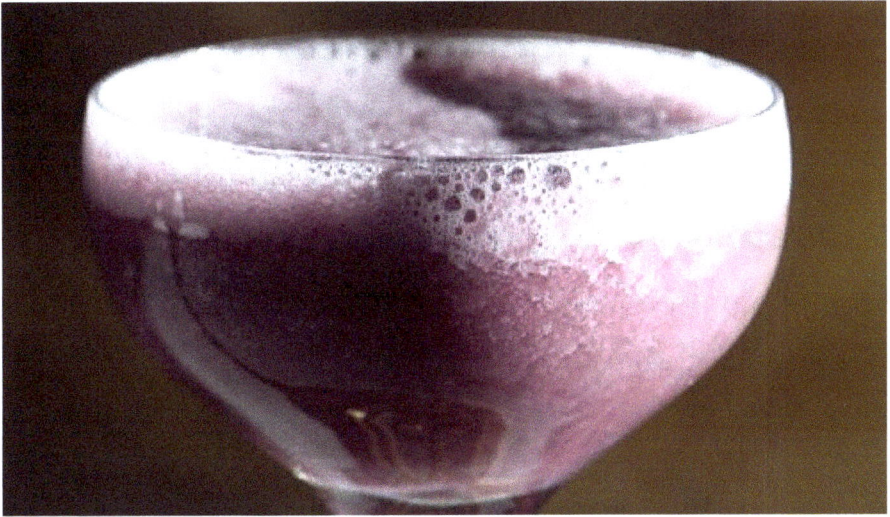

Gritty and Nutty Shake

Preparation time: 5 minutesCooking time: 0 minutes Servings: 1

Ingredients:

¼ cup heavy cream, liquid 1 tbsp almonds, sliced 1 tbsp macadamia nuts, whole 1 tbsp flaxseed 1 tbsp hemp seed What you'll need from the store cupboard: 1 packet Stevia, or more to taste 1 cup water ½ tbsp cocoa powder (optional) 3 tbsp coconut oil

Directions

Add all ingredients in a mixer. Whisk until smooth and creamy. Serve and enjoy

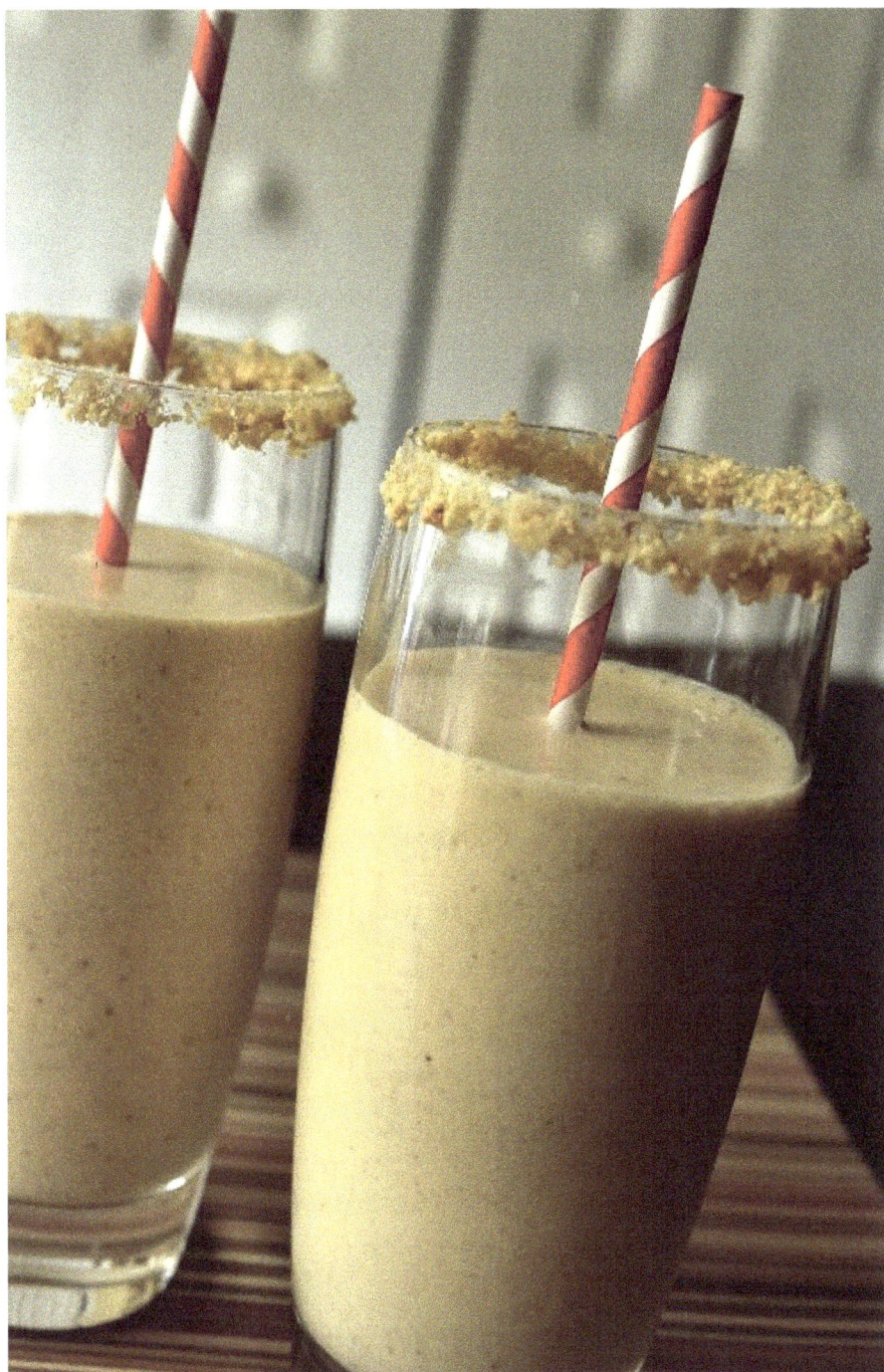

Warm Pomegranate Punch

Servings: 10 Preparation time: 2 hours and 15 minutes

Ingredients:

3 cinnamon sticks, each about 3 inches long 12 whole cloves 1/2 cup of coconut sugar 1/3 cup of lemon juice 32 fluid ounce of pomegranate juice 32 fluid ounce of apple juice, unsweetened 16 fluid ounce of brewed tea

Directions:

Using a 4-quart slow cooker, pour the lemon juice, pomegranate, juice apple juice, tea, and then sugar. Wrap the whole cloves and cinnamon stick in a cheese cloth, tie its corners with a string, and immerse it in the liquid present in the slow cooker. Then cover it with the lid, plug in the slow cooker and let it cook at the low heat setting for 3 hours or until it is heated thoroughly. When done, discard the cheesecloth bag and serve it hot or cold.

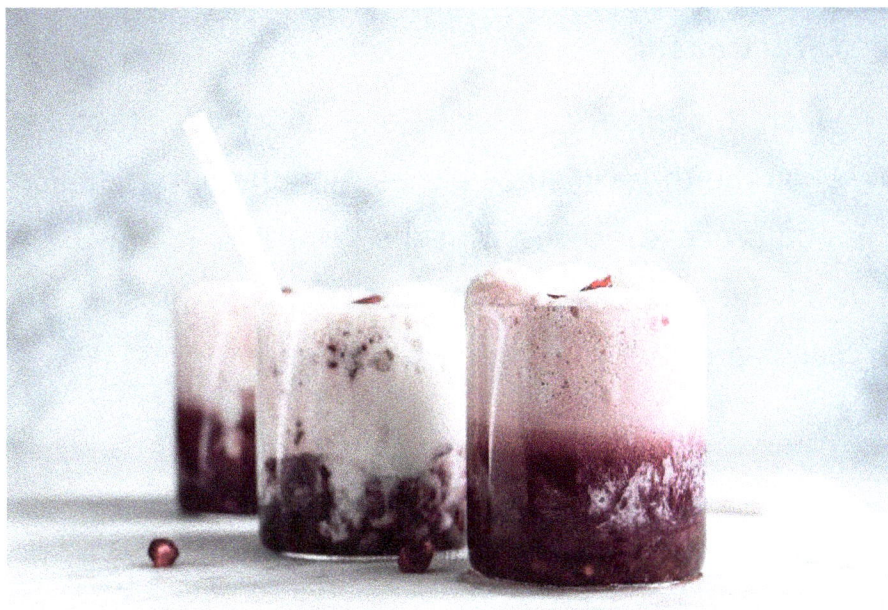

Apple and Cucumber Juice

Preparation time: 10 minutesCooking time: 0 minutes
Servings: 2

Ingredients:

3 apples 1 cucumber 2 celery stick 1 cup of vegetable milk Cinnamon, to taste Chia seeds (optional)

Directions:

Wash the apple, cucumber, and celery stick thoroughly. Chop the three in small pieces. Add them to the juicer or food processor along with the vegetable milk you chose and the cinnamon. If you wish to, top with some chia seeds and add a couple of ice cubes.

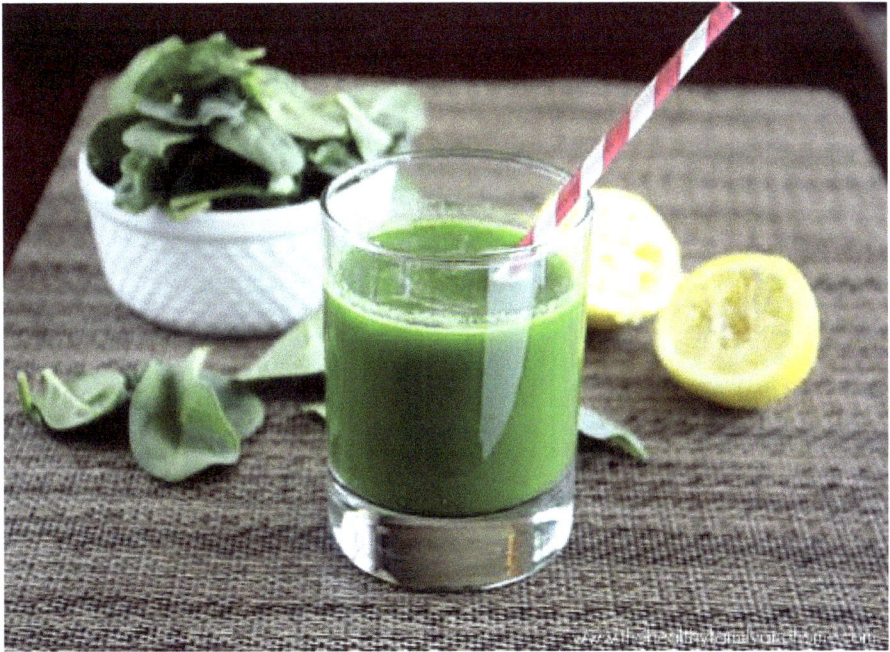

Minty-Coco and Greens Shake

Preparation time: 5 minutes Cooking time: 0 minutes Servings: 1

Ingredients:

½ cup coconut milk 2 peppermint leaves 2 packets Stevia, or as needed 1 cup 50/50 salad mix 1 tbsp coconut oil What you'll need from the store cupboard: 1 ½ cups water

Directions

Add all ingredients in a blender. Blend until smooth and creamy. Serve and enjoy.

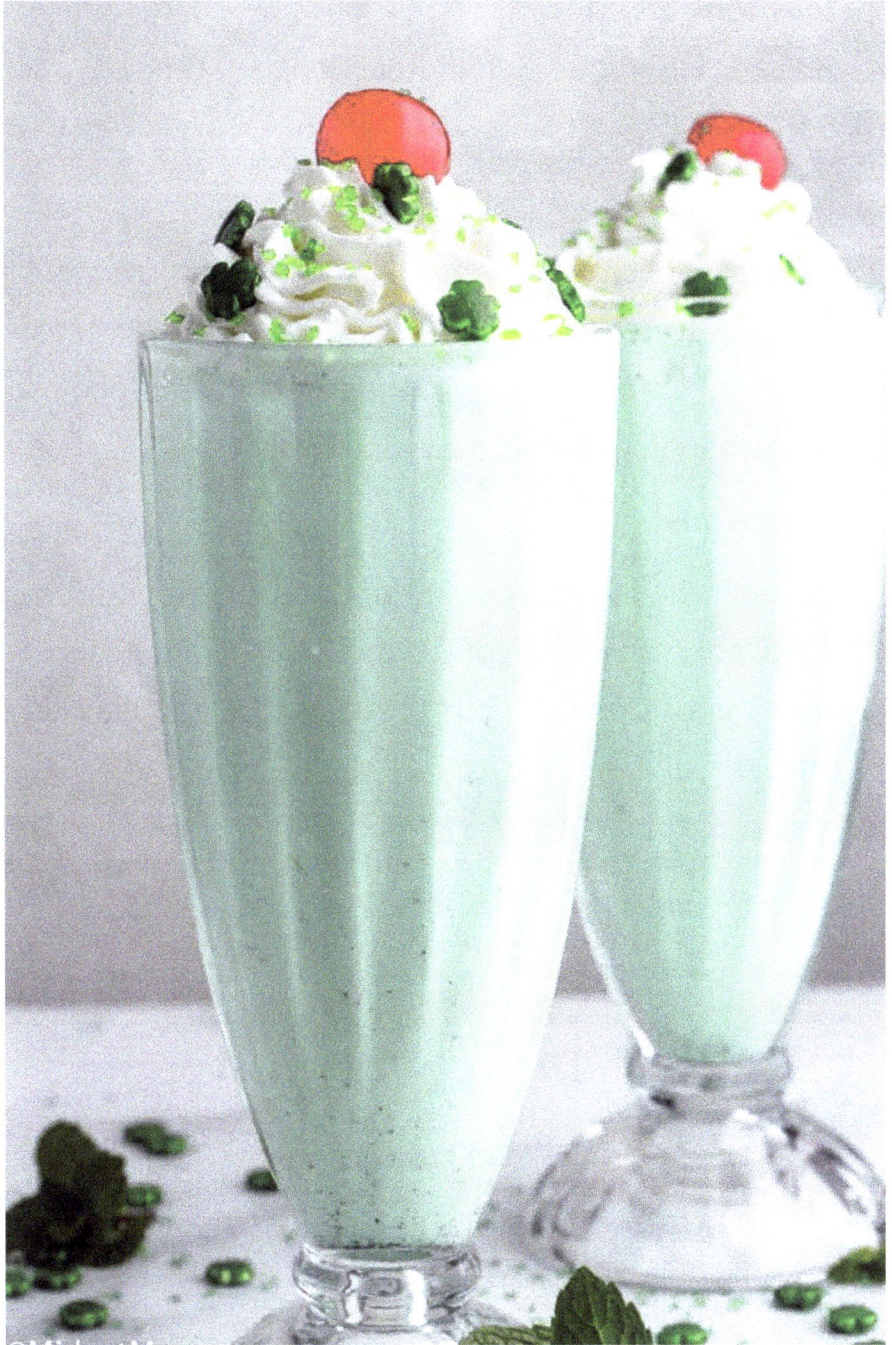

Turmeric Lassi

Preparation time: 5 minutes Cooking time: 0 minute Servings: 2

Ingredients:

1 teaspoon grated ginger 1/8 teaspoon ground black pepper 1 teaspoon turmeric powder 1/8 teaspoon cayenne 1 tablespoon coconut sugar 1/8 teaspoon salt 1 cup vegan yogurt 1 cup almond milk

Directions:

Place all the ingredients in the order in a food processor or blender and then pulse for 2 to 3 minutes at high speed until smooth. Pour the lassi into two glasses and then serve.

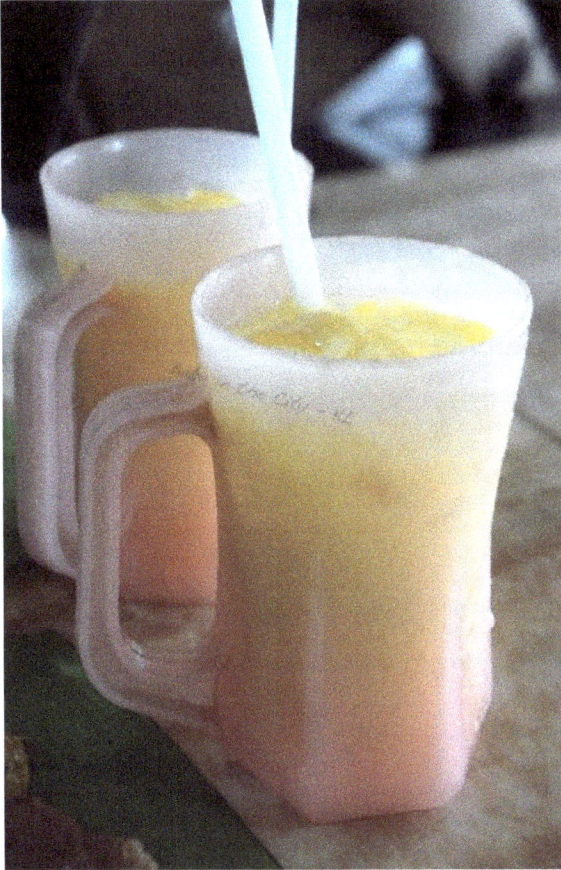

Saffron Pistachio Beverage

Preparation time: 5 minutes Cooking time: 0 minute Servings: 2

Ingredients:

8 strands of saffron 1 tablespoon cashews 1/4 teaspoon ground ginger 2 tablespoons pistachio 1/8 teaspoon cloves 1/4 teaspoon ground black pepper 1/4 teaspoon cardamom powder 3 tablespoons coconut sugar 1/4 teaspoon cinnamon 1/8 teaspoon fennel seeds 1/4 teaspoon poppy seeds

Directions:

Place all the ingredients in the order in a food processor or blender and then pulse for 2 to 3 minutes at high speed until smooth. Pour the smoothie into two glasses and then serve.

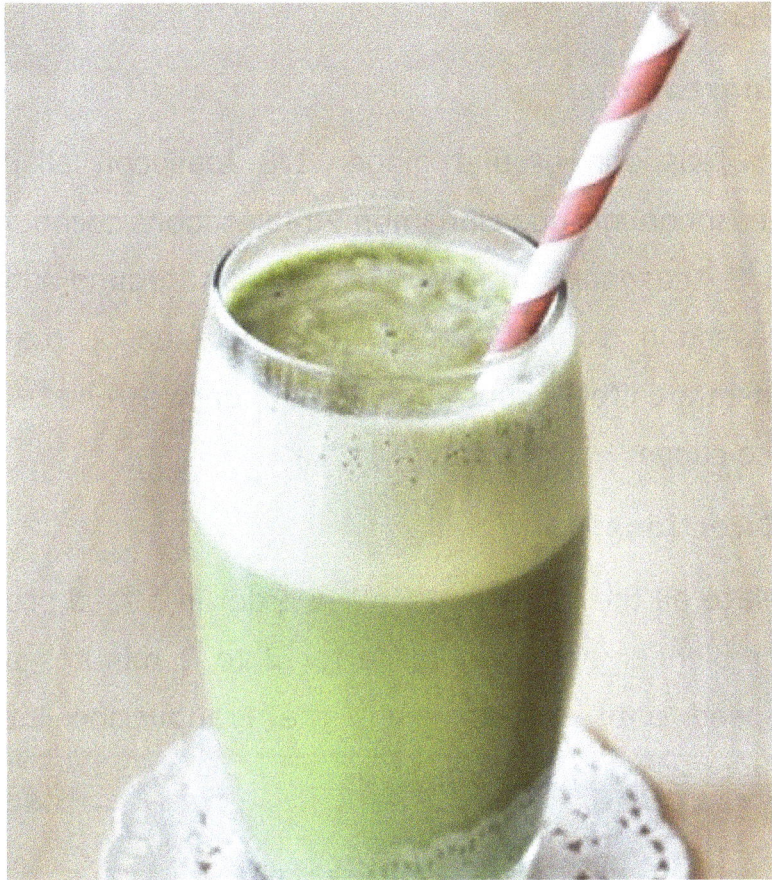

Pumpkin Spice Frappuccino

Preparation time: 5 minutes Cooking time: 0 minute Servings: 2

Ingredients:

½ teaspoon ground ginger 1/8 teaspoon allspice ½ teaspoon ground cinnamon 2 tablespoons coconut sugar 1/8 teaspoon nutmeg ¼ teaspoon ground cloves 1 teaspoon vanilla extract, unsweetened 2 teaspoons instant coffee 2 cups almond milk, unsweetened 1 cup of ice cubes

Directions:

Place all the ingredients in the order in a food processor or blender and then pulse for 2 to 3 minutes at high speed until smooth. Pour the Frappuccino into two glasses and then serve.

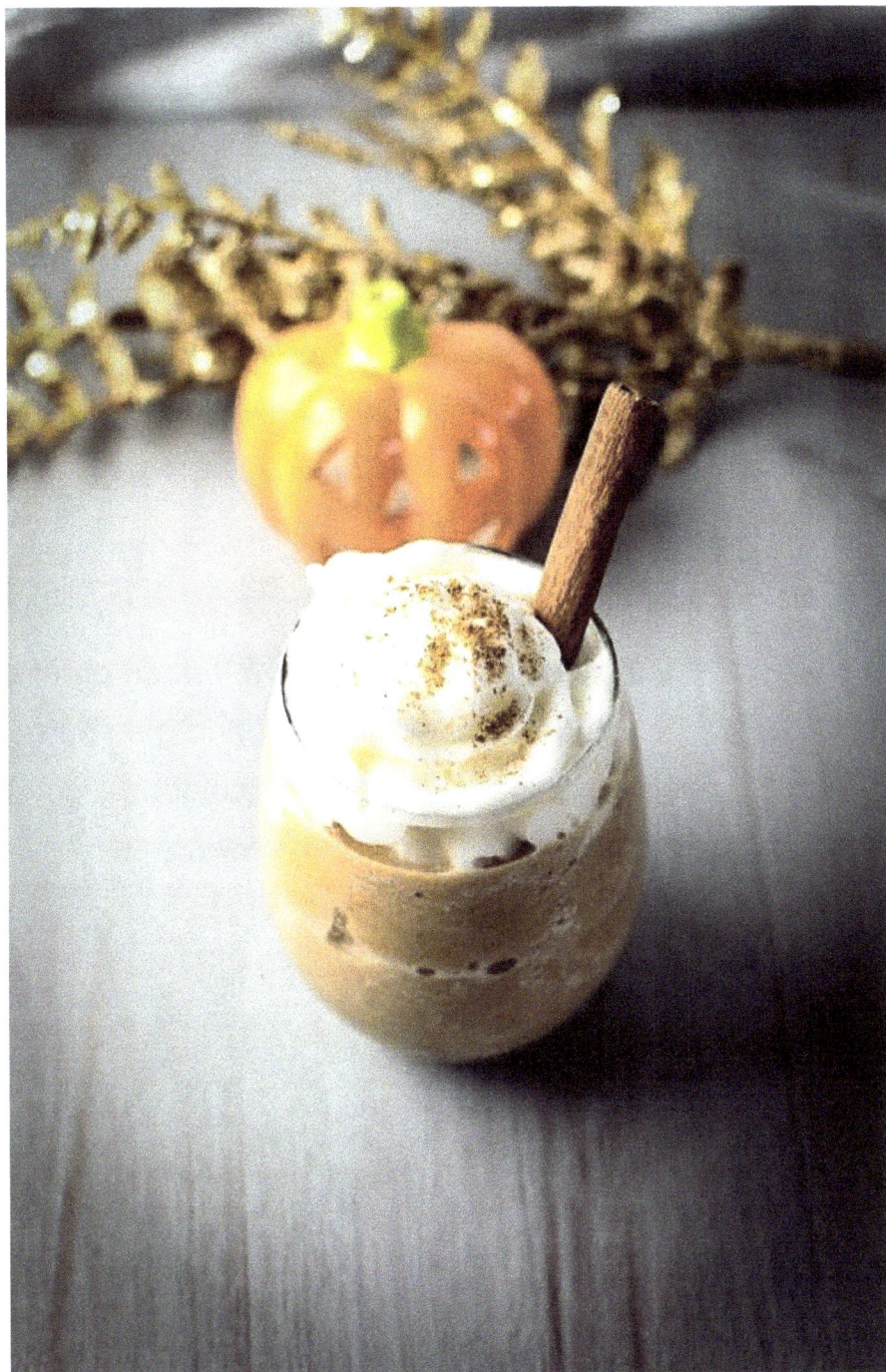

Strawberry and Hemp Smoothie

Preparation time: 5 minutes Cooking time: 0 minute Servings: 2

Ingredients:

3 cups fresh strawberries 2 tablespoons hemp seeds 1/2 teaspoon vanilla extract, unsweetened 1/8 teaspoon sea salt 2 tablespoons maple syrup 1 cup vegan yogurt 1 cup almond milk, unsweetened 1 cup of ice cubes 2 tablespoons hemp protein

Directions:

Place all the ingredients in the order in a food processor or blender, except for protein powder, and then pulse for 2 to 3 minutes at high speed until smooth. Pour the smoothie into two glasses and then serve.

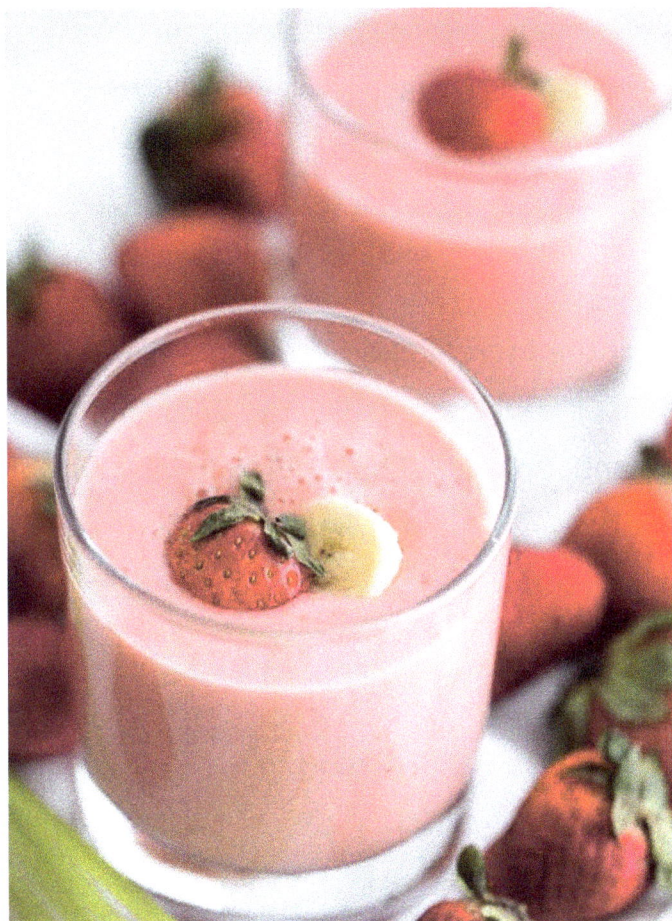

Mango Lassi

Preparation time: 5 minutes Cooking time: 0 minute Servings: 2

Ingredients:

1 ¼ cup mango pulp 1 tablespoon coconut sugar 1/8 teaspoon salt 1/2 teaspoon lemon juice 1/4 cup almond milk, unsweetened 1/4 cup chilled water 1 cup cashew yogurt

Directions:

Place all the ingredients in the order in a food processor or blender and then pulse for 2 to 3 minutes at high speed until smooth. Pour the lassi into two glasses and then serve.

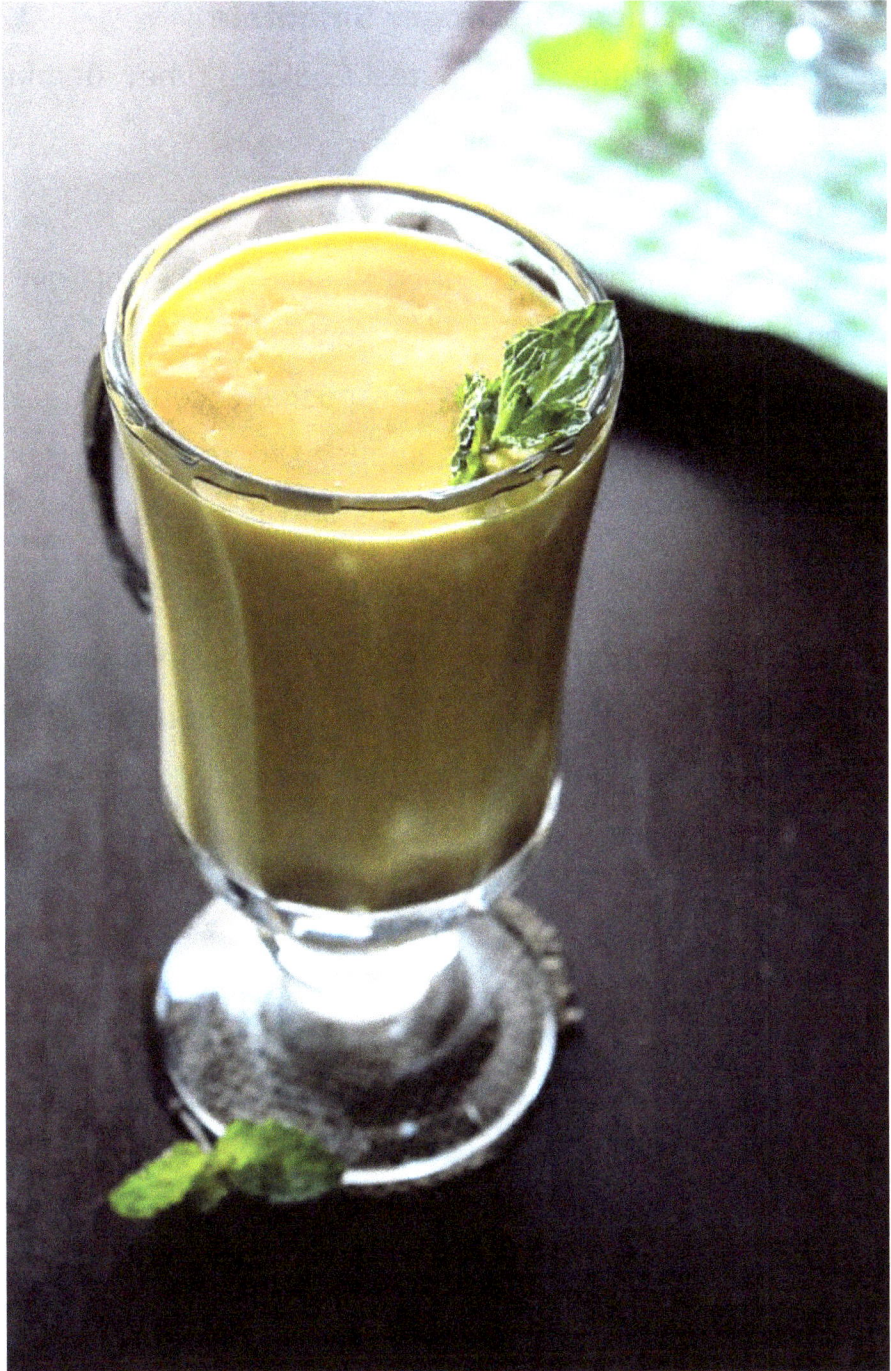

Chard, Lettuce and Ginger Smoothie

Preparation time: 5 minutes Cooking time: 0 minute Servings: 2

Ingredients:

10 Chard leaves, chopped 1-inch piece of ginger, chopped 10 lettuce leaves, chopped ½ teaspoon black salt 2 pear, chopped 2 teaspoons coconut sugar ¼ teaspoon ground black pepper ¼ teaspoon salt 2 tablespoons lemon juice 2 cups of water

Directions:

Place all the ingredients in the order in a food processor or blender and then pulse for 2 to 3 minutes at high speed until smooth. Pour the smoothie into two glasses and then serve.

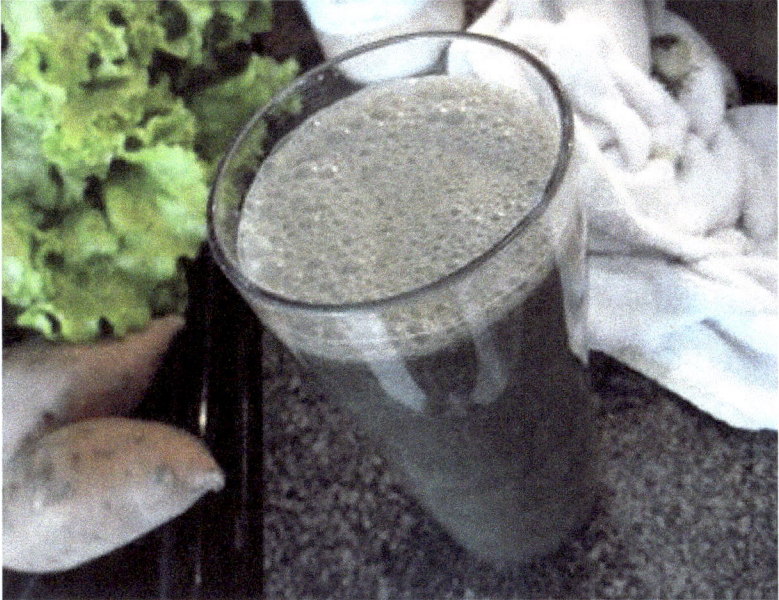

Berry and Yogurt Smoothie

Preparation time: 5 minutes Cooking time: 0 minute Servings: 2

Ingredients:

2 small bananas 3 cups frozen mixed berries 1 ½ cup cashew yogurt 1/2 teaspoon vanilla extract, unsweetened 1/2 cup almond milk, unsweetened

Directions:

Place all the ingredients in the order in a food processor or blender and then pulse for 2 to 3 minutes at high speed until smooth. Pour the smoothie into two glasses and then serve.

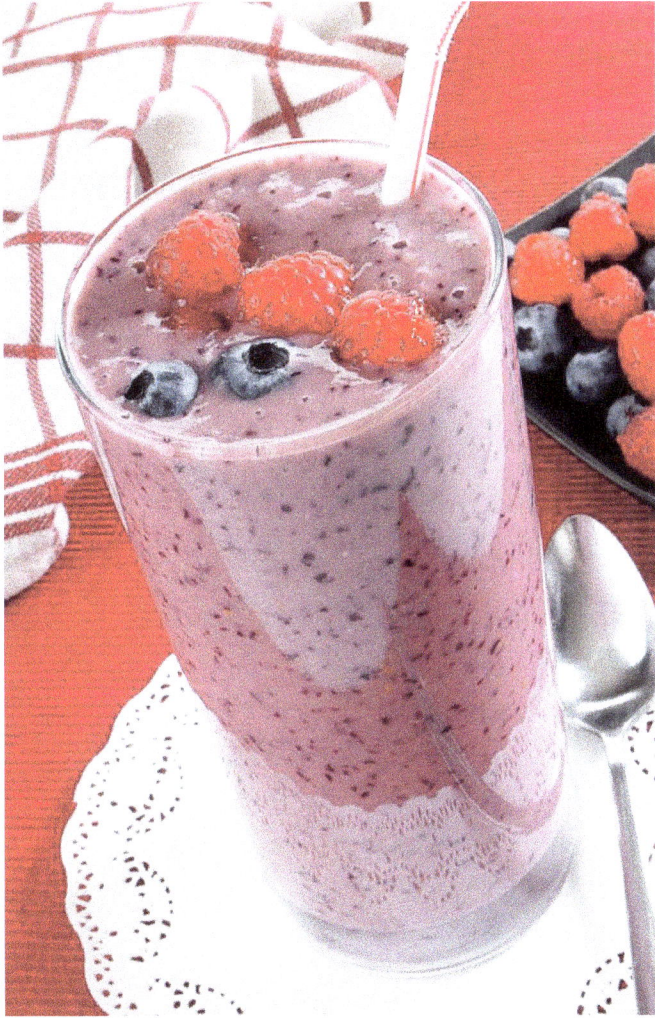

Strawberry and Chocolate Milkshake

Preparation time: 5 minutes Cooking time: 0 minute Servings: 2

Ingredients:

2 cups frozen strawberries 3 tablespoons cocoa powder 1 scoop protein powder 2 tablespoons maple syrup 1 teaspoon vanilla extract, unsweetened 2 cups almond milk, unsweetened

Directions:

Place all the ingredients in the order in a food processor or blender and then pulse for 2 to 3 minutes at high speed until smooth. Pour the smoothie into two glasses and then serve.

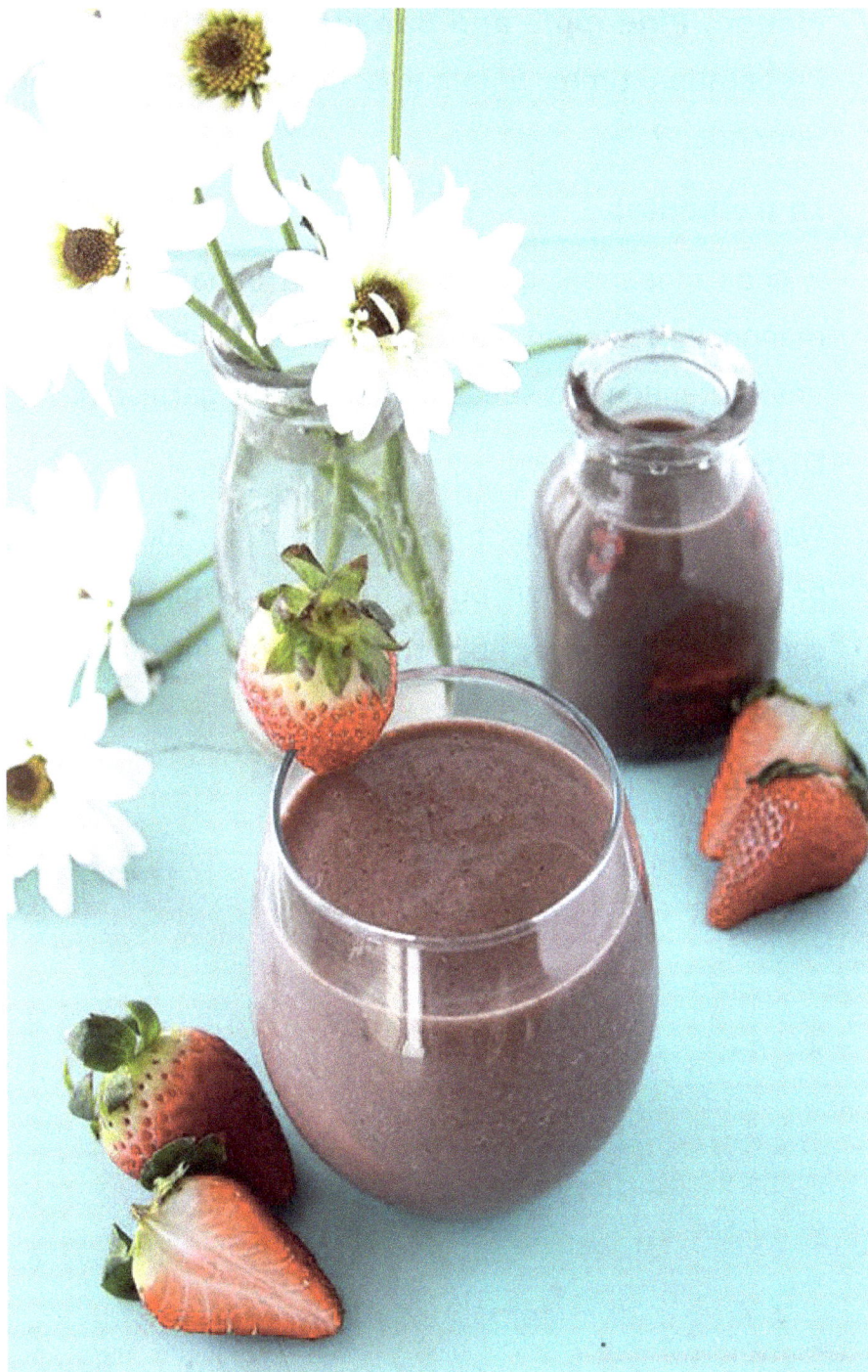

Mango, Pineapple and Banana Smoothie

Preparation time: 5 minutes Cooking time: 0 minute Servings: 2

Ingredients:

2 cups pineapple chunks 2 frozen bananas 2 medium mangoes, destoned, cut into chunks 1 cup almond milk, unsweetened Chia seeds as needed for garnishing

Directions:

Place all the ingredients in the order in a food processor or blender and then pulse for 2 to 3 minutes at high speed until smooth. Pour the smoothie into two glasses and then serve.

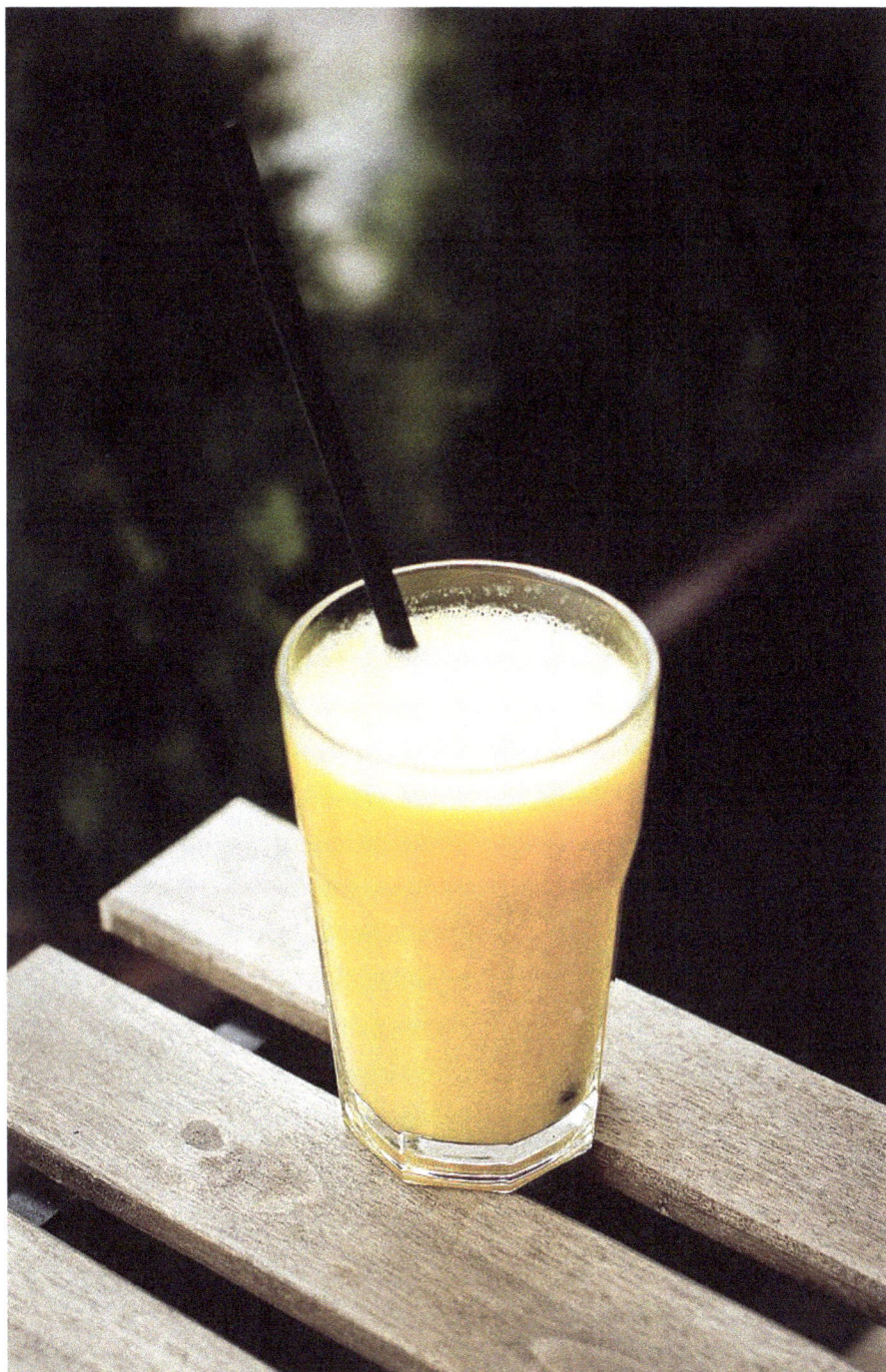

Spiced Buttermilk

Preparation time: 5 minutes Cooking time: 0 minute Servings: 2

Ingredients:

3/4 teaspoon ground cumin 1/4 teaspoon sea salt 1/8 teaspoon ground black pepper 2 mint leaves 1/8 teaspoon lemon juice ¼ cup cilantro leaves 1 cup of chilled water 1 cup vegan yogurt, unsweetened Ice as needed

Directions:

Place all the ingredients in the order in a food processor or blender, except for cilantro and ¼ teaspoon cumin, and then pulse for 2 to 3 minutes at high speed until smooth. Pour the milk into glasses, top with cilantro and cumin, and then serve.

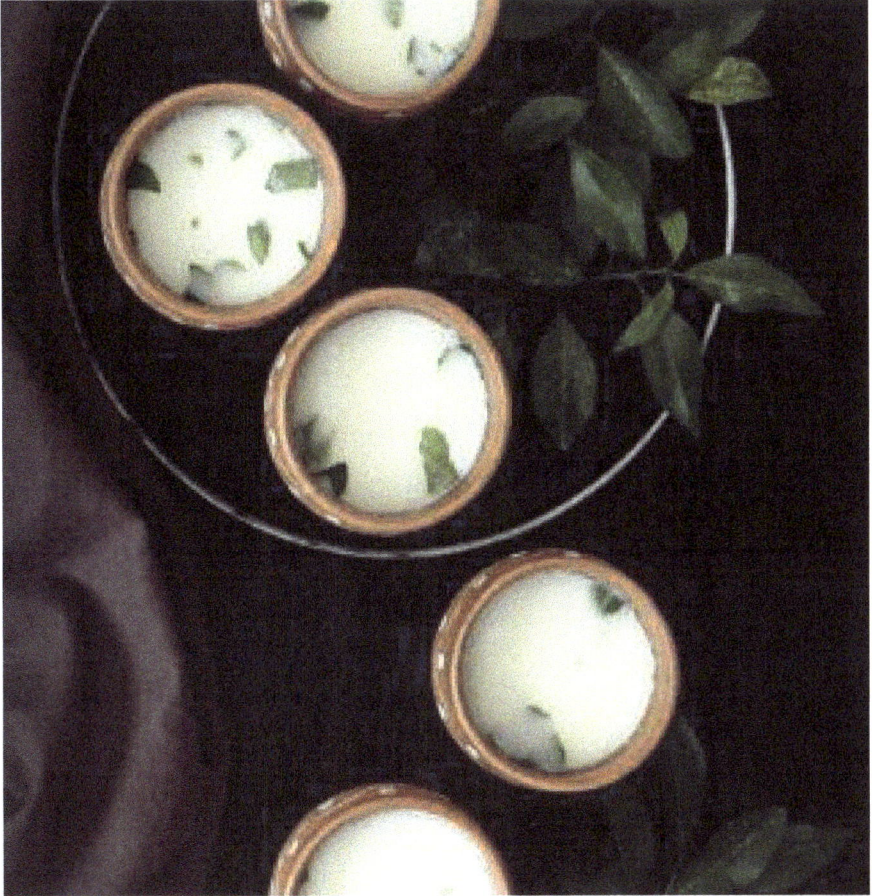

Brownie Batter Orange Chia Shake

Preparation time: 5 minutes Cooking time: 0 minute
Servings: 2

Ingredients:

2 tablespoons cocoa powder 3 tablespoons chia seeds ¼ teaspoon salt 4 tablespoons chocolate chips 4 teaspoons coconut sugar ½ teaspoon orange zest ½ teaspoon vanilla extract, unsweetened 2 cup almond milk

Directions:

Place all the ingredients in the order in a food processor or blender and then pulse for 2 to 3 minutes at high speed until smooth. Pour the smoothie into two glasses and then serve.

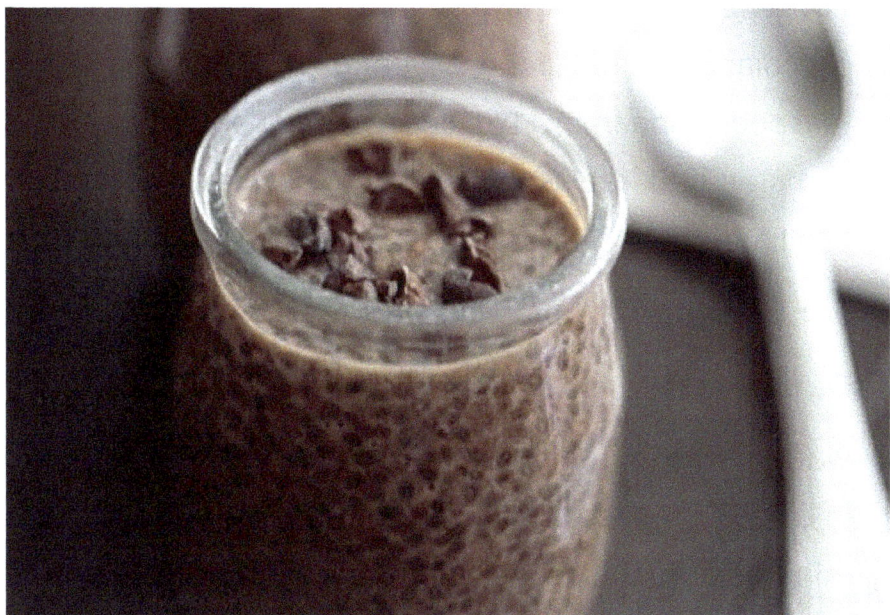

Mexican Hot Chocolate Mix

Preparation time: 5 minutes Cooking time: 0 minute Servings: 2

Ingredients:

For the Hot Chocolate Mix: 1/3 cup chopped dark chocolate 1/8 teaspoon cayenne 1/8 teaspoon salt 1/2 teaspoon cinnamon 1/4 cup coconut sugar 1 teaspoon cornstarch 3 tablespoons cocoa powder 1/2 teaspoon vanilla extract, unsweetened

For Serving: 2 cups milk, warmed

Directions:

Place all the ingredients of hot chocolate mix in the order in a food processor or blender and then pulse for 2 to 3 minutes at high speed until ground. Stir 2 tablespoons of the chocolate mix into a glass of milk until combined and then serve

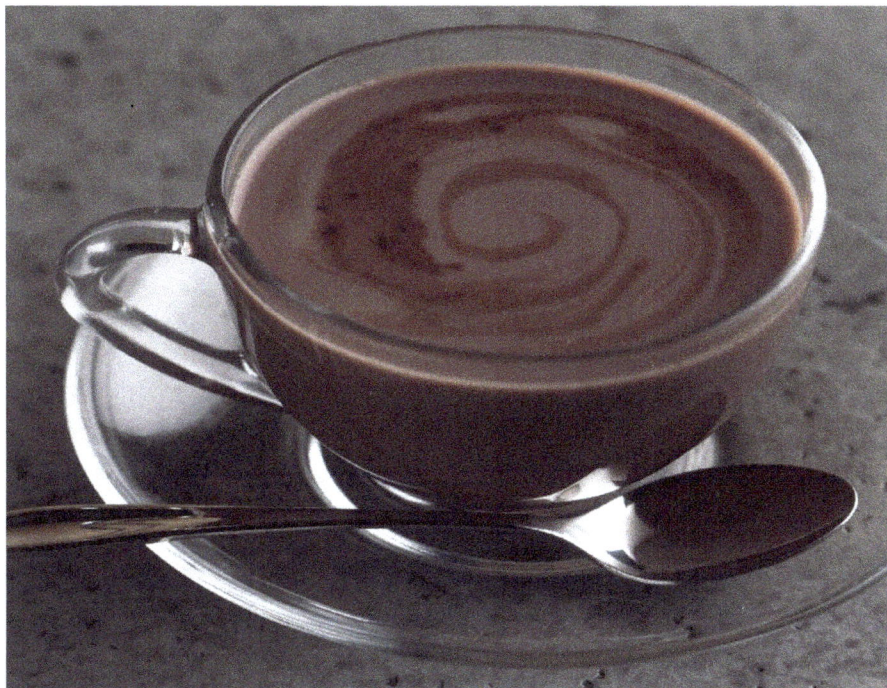

Cookie Dough Milkshake

Preparation time: 5 minutes Cooking time: 0 minute Servings: 2

Ingredients:

2 tablespoons cookie dough 5 dates, pitted 2 teaspoons chocolate chips 1/2 teaspoon vanilla extract, unsweetened 1/2 cup almond milk, unsweetened 1 ½ cup almond milk ice cubes

Directions:

Place all the ingredients in the order in a food processor or blender and then pulse for 2 to 3 minutes at high speed until smooth. Pour the milkshake into two glasses and then serve with some cookie dough balls.

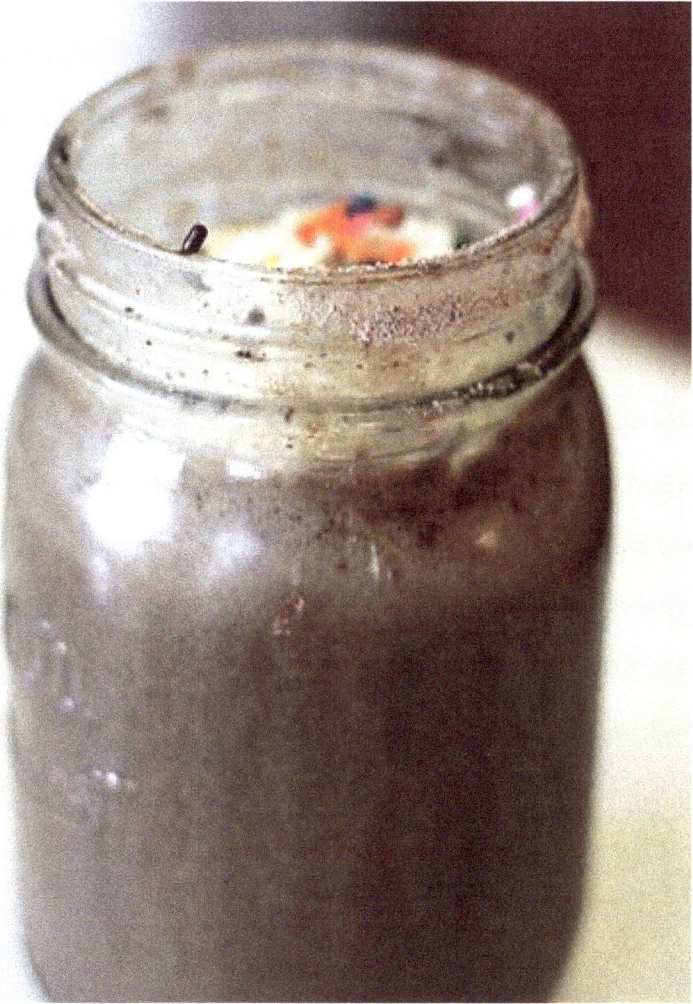

Blueberry, Hazelnut and Hemp Smoothie

Preparation time: 5 minutes Cooking time: 0 minute Servings: 2

Ingredients:

2 tablespoons hemp seeds 1 ½ cups frozen blueberries 2 tablespoons chocolate protein powder 1/2 teaspoon vanilla extract, unsweetened 2 tablespoons chocolate hazelnut butter 1 small frozen banana 3/4 cup almond milk

Directions:

Place all the ingredients in the order in a food processor or blender and then pulse for 2 to 3 minutes at high speed until smooth. Pour the smoothie into two glasses and then serve.

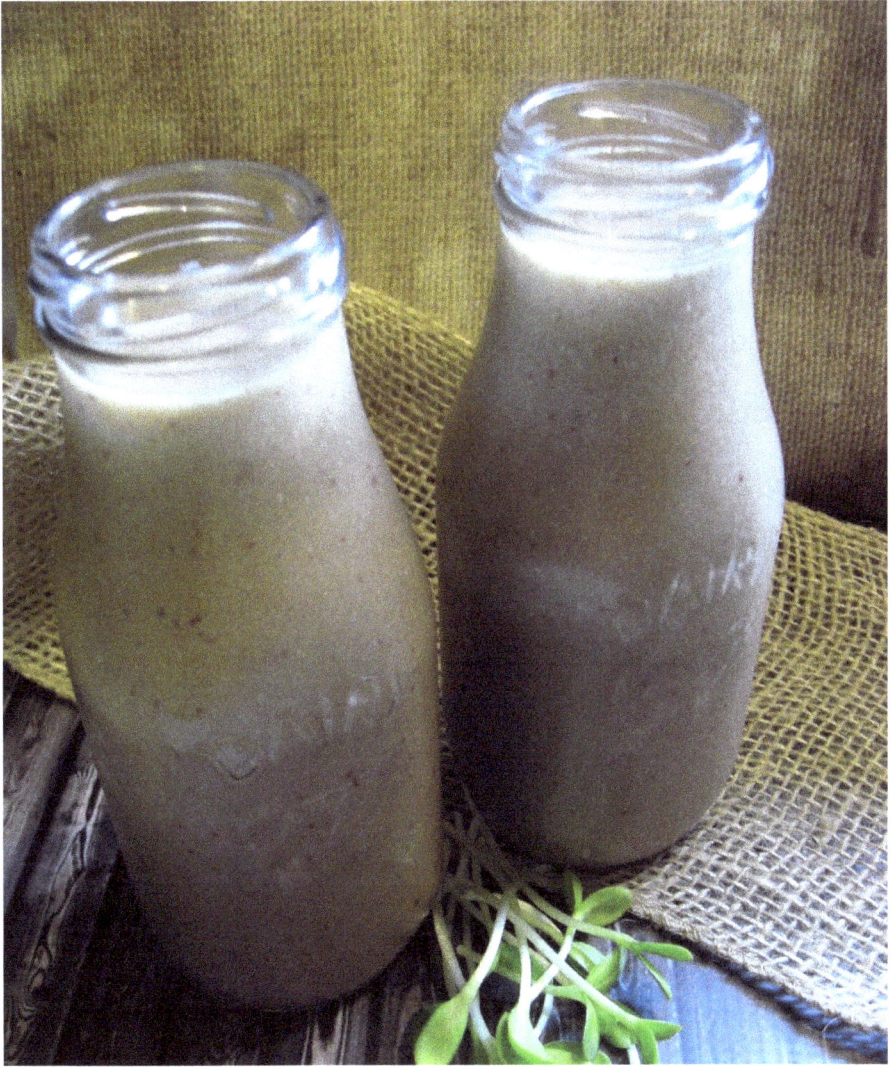

Mocha Chocolate Shake

Preparation time: 5 minutes Cooking time: 0 minute Servings: 2

Ingredients:

1/4 cup hemp seeds 2 teaspoons cocoa powder, unsweetened 1/2 cup dates, pitted 1 tablespoon instant coffee powder 2 tablespoons flax seeds 2 1/2 cups almond milk, unsweetened 1/2 cup crushed ice

Directions:

Place all the ingredients in the order in a food processor or blender and then pulse for 2 to 3 minutes at high speed until smooth. Pour the smoothie into two glasses and then serve.

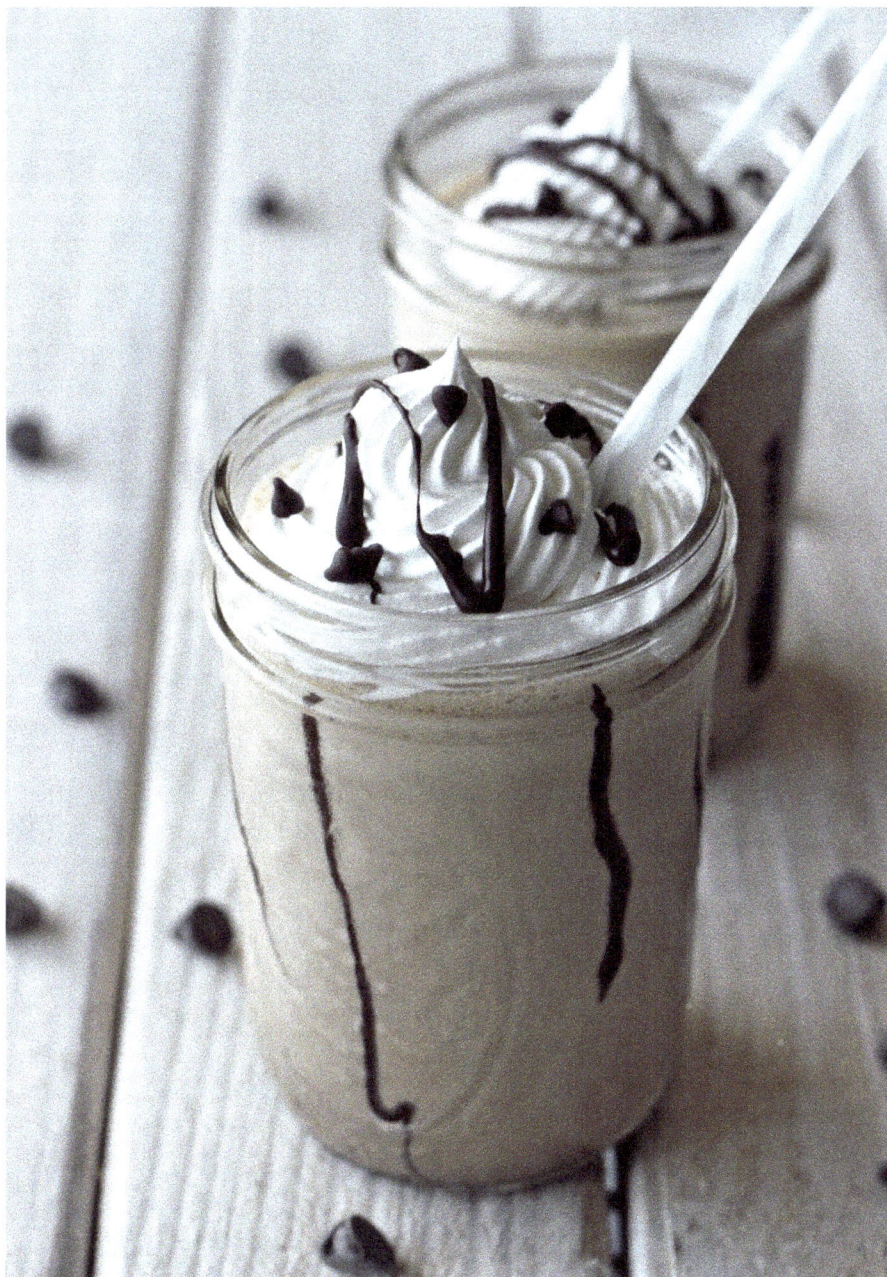

Red Beet, Pear and Apple Smoothie

Preparation time: 5 minutes Cooking time: 0 minute

Servings: 2

Ingredients:

1/2 of medium beet, peeled, chopped 1 tablespoon chopped cilantro 1 orange, juiced 1 medium pear, chopped 1 medium apple, cored, chopped 1/4 teaspoon ground black pepper 1/8 teaspoon rock salt 1 teaspoon coconut sugar 1/4 teaspoons salt 1 cup of water

Directions:

Place all the ingredients in the order in a food processor or blender and then pulse for 2 to 3 minutes at high speed until smooth. Pour the smoothie into two glasses and then serve.

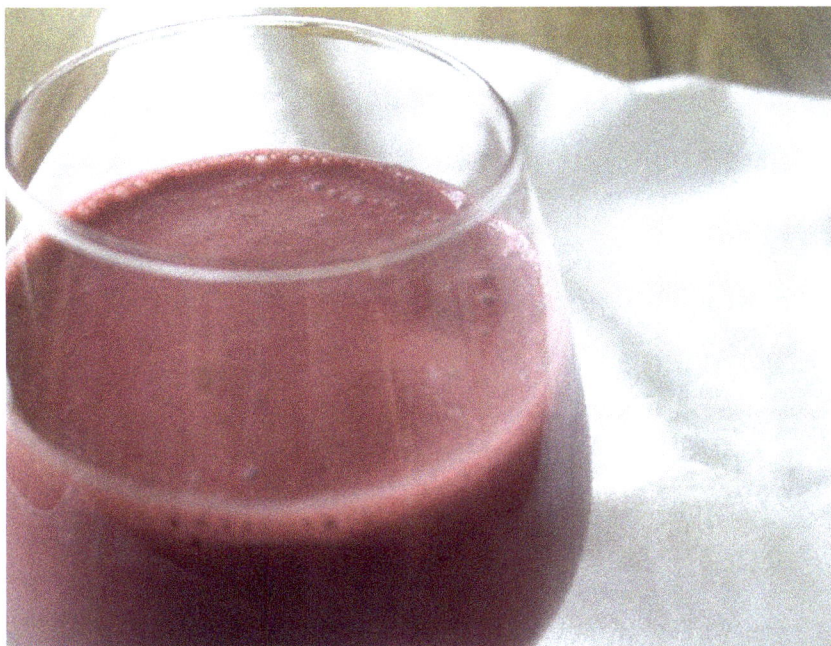

Chocolate and Cherry Smoothie

Preparation time: 5 minutes Cooking time: 0 minute Servings: 2

Ingredients:

4 cups frozen cherries 2 tablespoons cocoa powder 1 scoop of protein powder 1 teaspoon maple syrup 2 cups almond milk, unsweetened

Directions:

Place all the ingredients in the order in a food processor or blender and then pulse for 2 to 3 minutes at high speed until smooth. Pour the smoothie into two glasses and then serve.

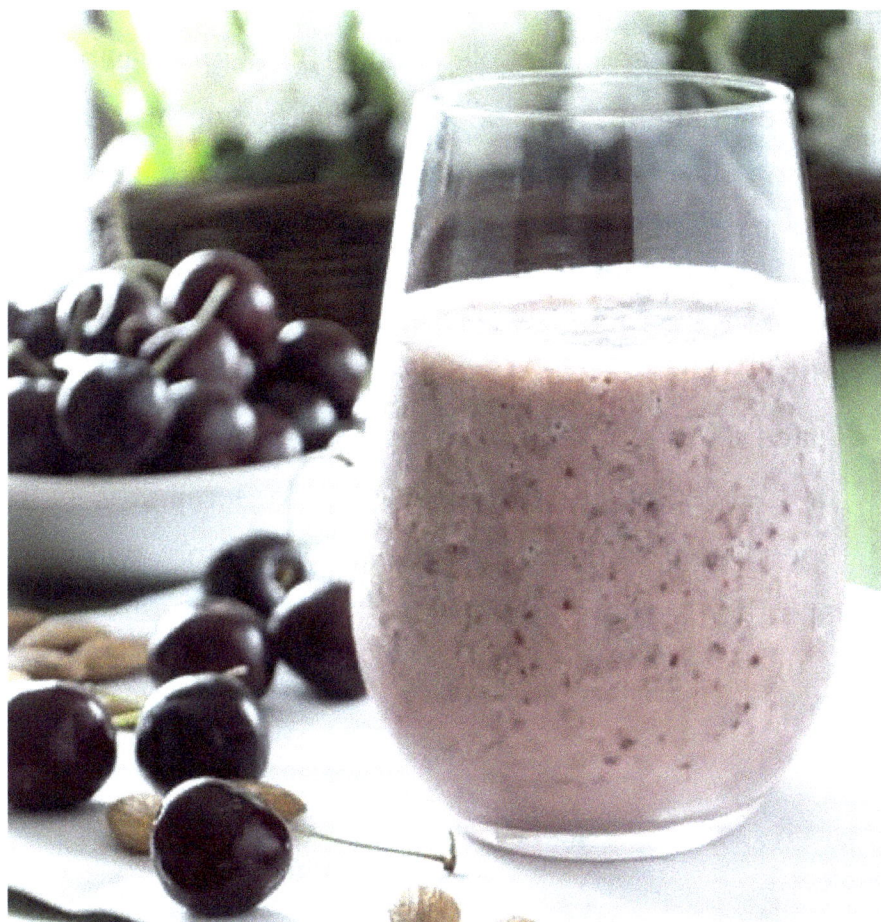

Banana and Protein Smoothie

Preparation time: 5 minutes Cooking time: 0 minute Servings: 2

Ingredients:

2/3 cup frozen pineapple chunk 10 frozen strawberries 2 frozen bananas 2 scoops protein powder 2 teaspoons cocoa powder 2 tablespoons maple syrup 2 teaspoons vanilla extract, unsweetened 2 cups almond milk, unsweetened

Directions:

Place all the ingredients in the order in a food processor or blender and then pulse for 2 to 3 minutes at high speed until smooth. Pour the smoothie into two glasses and then serve.

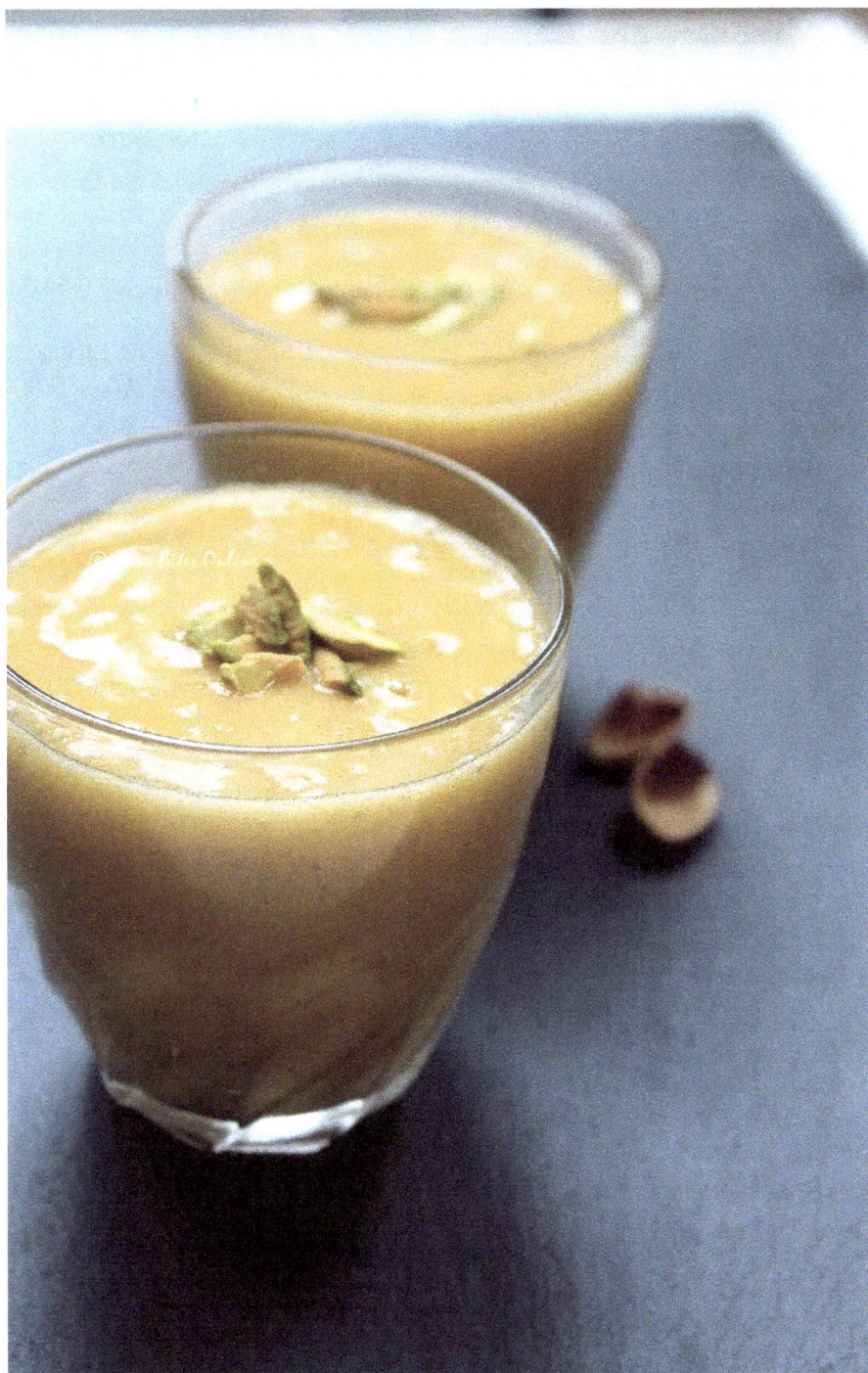

Blueberry and Banana Smoothie

Preparation time: 5 minutes Cooking time: 0 minute Servings: 2

Ingredients:

2 frozen bananas 2 cups frozen blueberries 2 cups almond milk, unsweetened 1/2 teaspoon or so cinnamon dash of vanilla extract

Directions:

Place all the ingredients in the order in a food processor or blender and then pulse for 2 to 3 minutes at high speed until smooth. Pour the smoothie into two glasses and then serve.

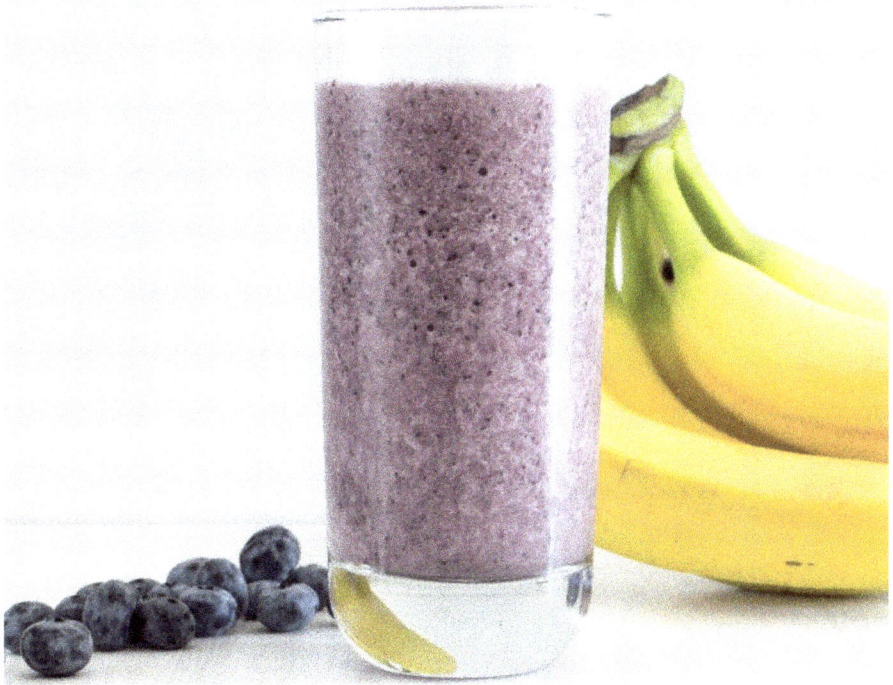

Miami Mango Shake

Preparation time: 30 minutes Cooking time: 0 minutes Servings: 01

Ingredients:

1 cup unsweetened coconut milk 1 scoop protein powder 1 cup frozen mango 1 cup frozen strawberries

Directions:

Add all ingredients to a blender. Hit the pulse button and blend till it is smooth. Chill well to serve.

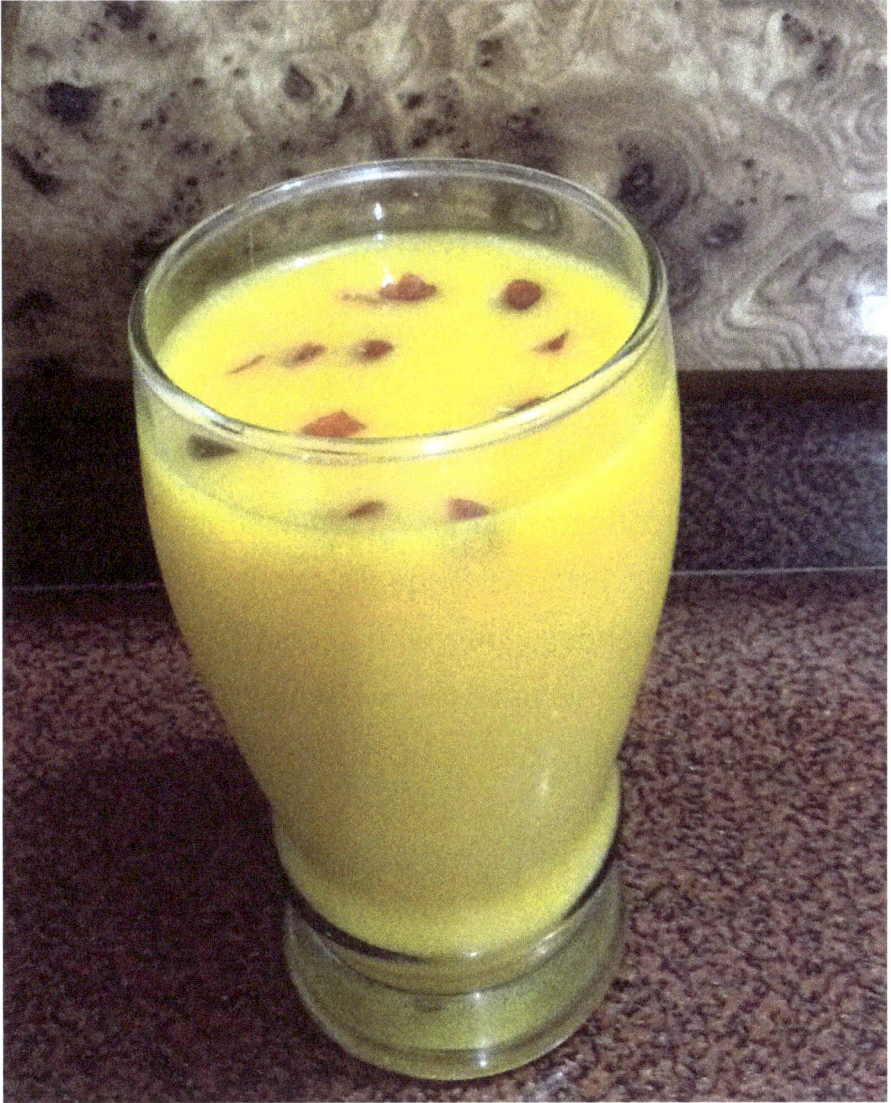

Iced Tea

Preparation time: 5 minutes Cooking time: 0 minutes Servings: 2

Ingredients:

A cup high quality tea bag A tablespoon of coconut butter A tablespoon of plant-based milk of your choice Optional add-ins: 1 teaspoon of MCT oil 1 teaspoon of cinnamon 1 teaspoon of vanilla powder 1 teaspoon of coconut milk powder (instead of the plant milk)

Directions:

Brew your coffee – either a French press or automatic coffee maker using high-quality coffee. Add a cup of coffee in a blender along with coconut butter and other add-ins and blend until foamy. Pour in a mug and top with foamed plant milk or dust with cinnamon.

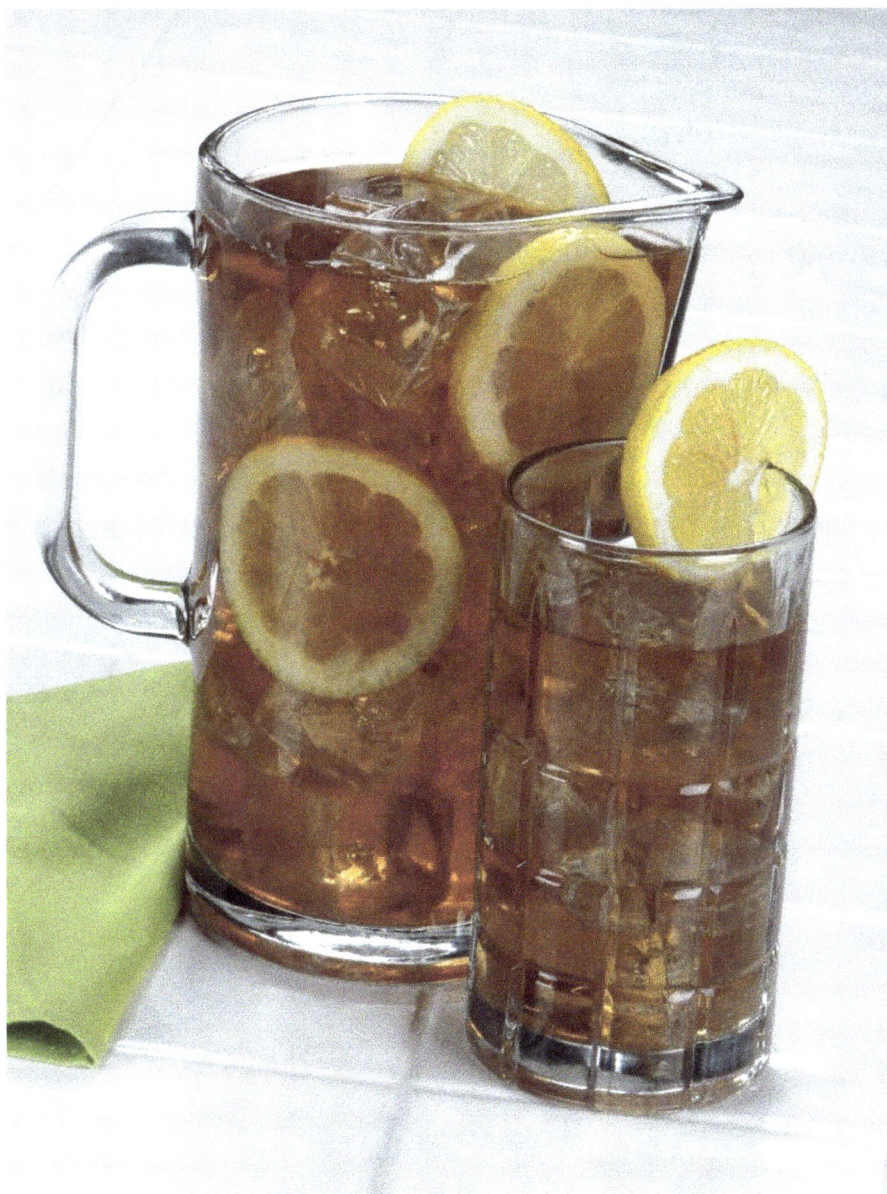

Strawberry-Choco Shake

Preparation time: 5 minutes Cooking time: 0 minutes Servings: 1

Ingredients:

½ cup heavy cream, liquid 1 tbsp cocoa powder 1 packet Stevia, or more to taste 4 strawberries, sliced 1 tbsp coconut flakes, unsweetened What you'll need from the store cupboard: 1 ½ cups water 3 tbsps coconut oil

Directions

Add all ingredients in a blender. Blend until smooth and creamy. Serve and enjoy.

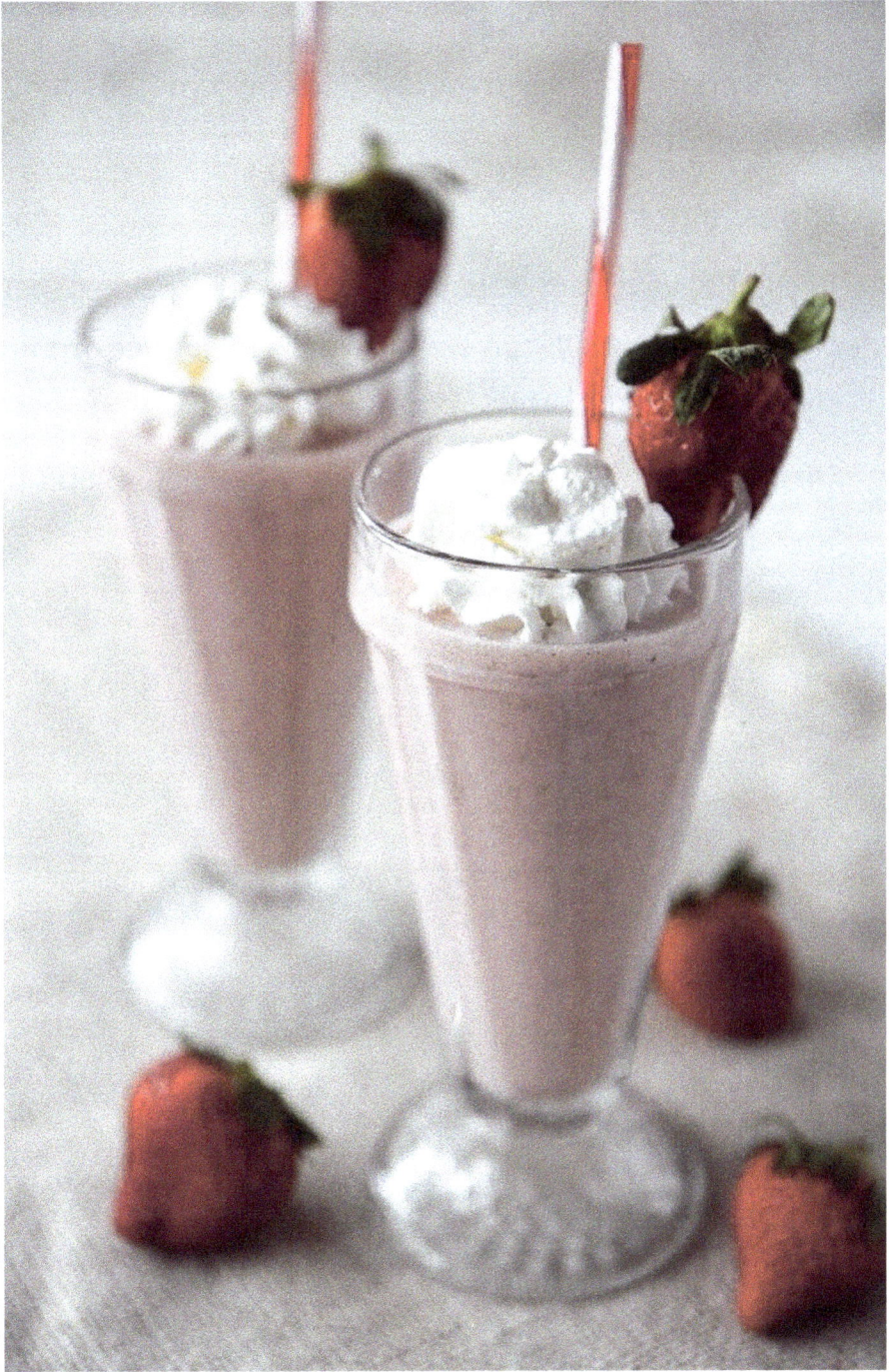

Creamy Choco Shake

Preparation time: 5 minutes Cooking time: 0 minutes Servings: 1

Ingredients:

½ cup heavy cream 2 tbsp cocoa powder 1 packet Stevia, or more to taste 1 cup water What you'll need from the store cupboard: 3 tbsps coconut oil

Directions Add all ingredients in a blender. Blend until smooth and creamy. Serve and enjoy.

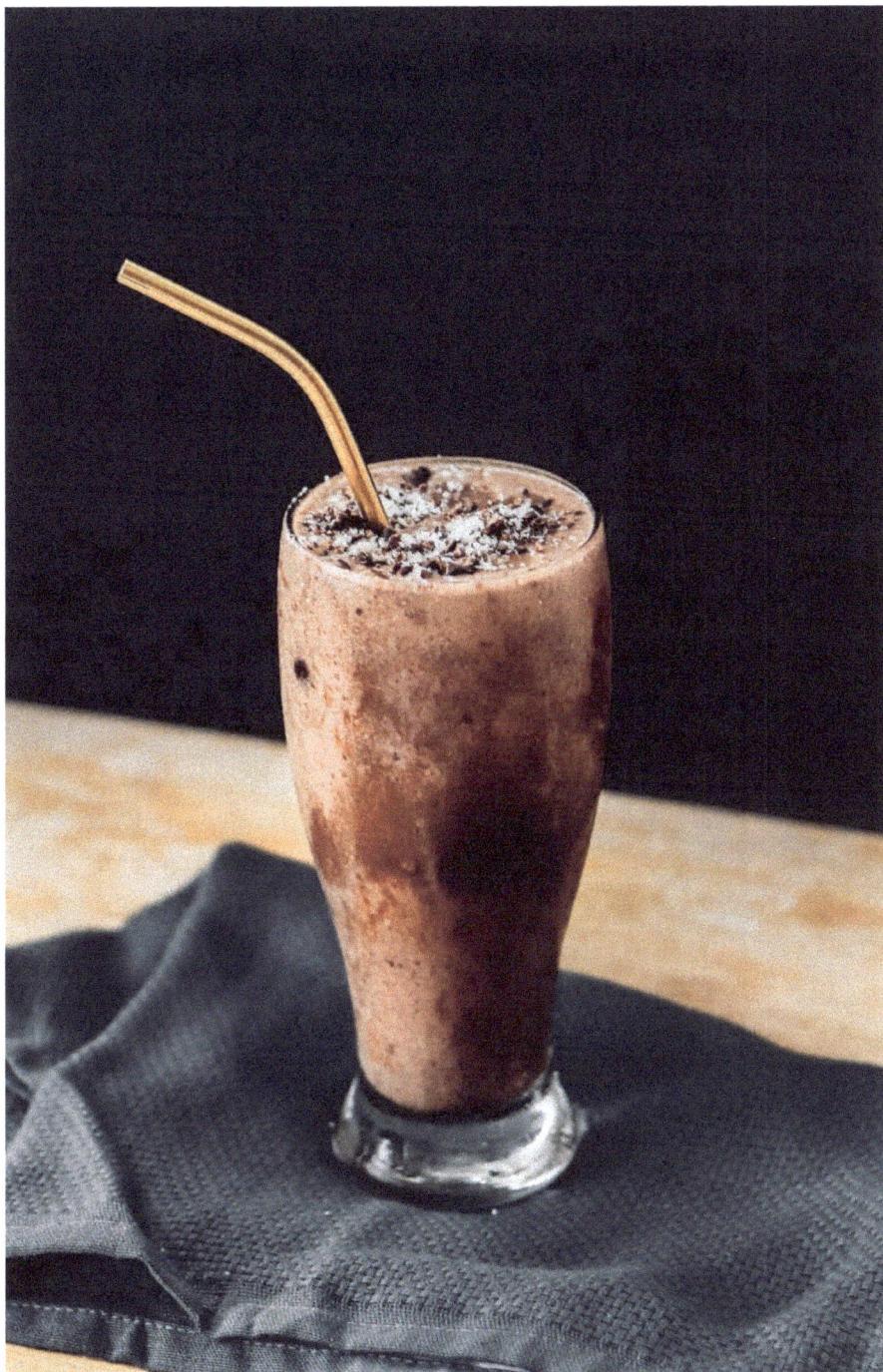

No Cook Coconut and Chocolate Bars

Preparation time: 15 minutesCooking time: 0 minutes

Servings: 6

Ingredients:

1 tbsp Stevia ¾ cup shredded coconut, unsweetened ½ cup ground nuts (almonds, pecans, or walnuts) ¼ cup unsweetened cocoa powder 4 tbsp coconut oil What you'll need from the store cupboard: Done

Directions In a medium bowl, mix shredded coconut, nuts, and cocoa powder. Add Stevia and coconut oil. Mix batter thoroughly. In a 9x9 square inch pan or dish, press the batter and for a 30-minutes place in the freezer. Serve and enjoy.

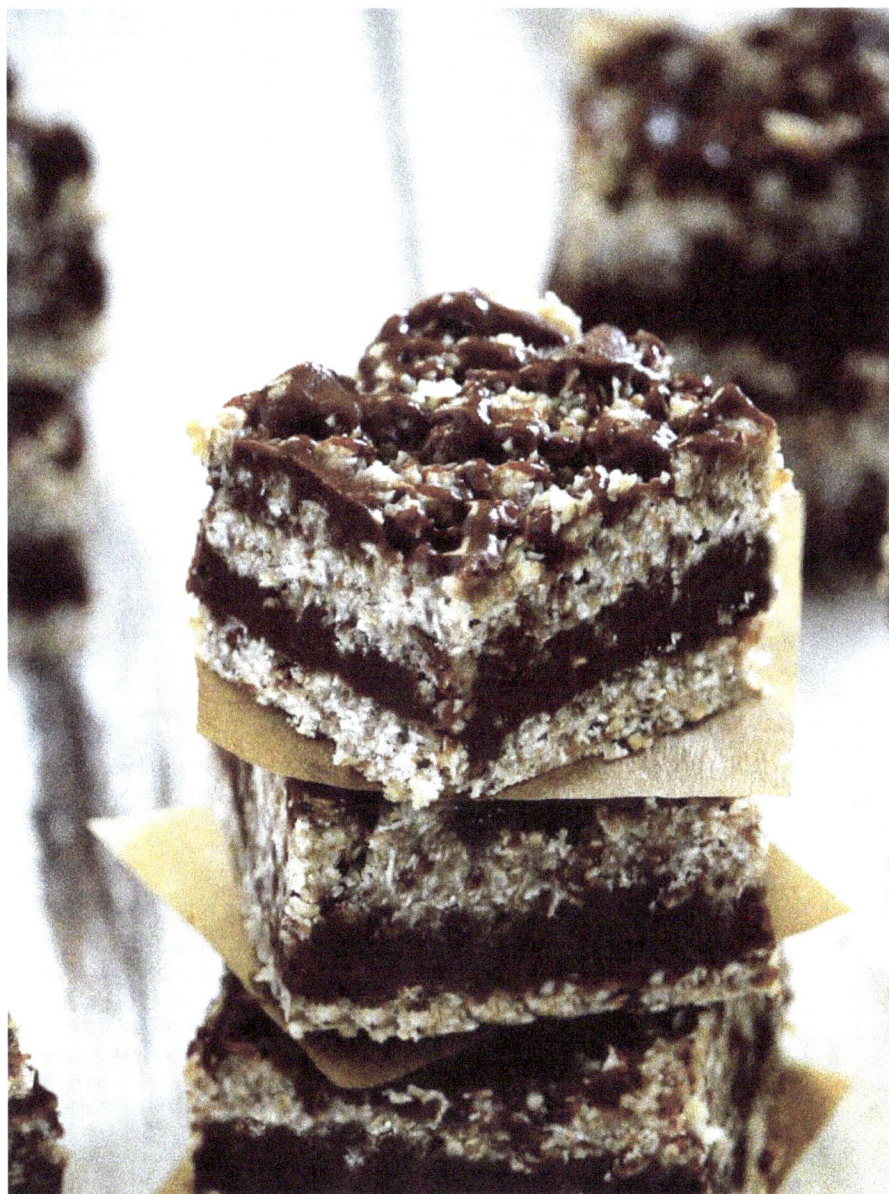

Chocolate Mousse

Preparation time: 15 minutesCooking time: 0 minutes
Servings: 4

Ingredients:

1 large, ripe avocado 1/4 cup sweetened almond milk 1 tbsp coconut oil 1/4 cup cocoa or cacao powder 1 tsp vanilla extract What you'll need from the store cupboard: none

Directions In a food processor, process all ingredients until smooth and creamy. Transfer to a lidded container and chill for at least 4 hours. Serve and enjoy.

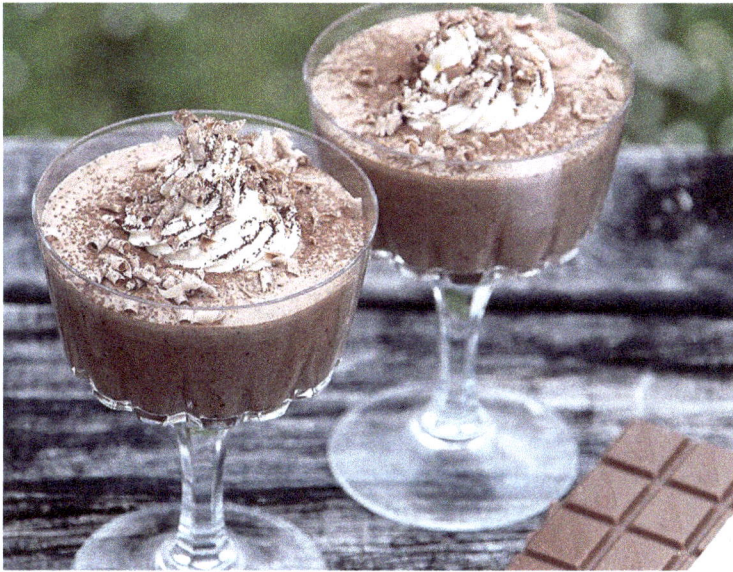

Apple Tart

Preparation time: 5 minutesCooking time: 40 minutes

Servings: 4

Ingredients:

crust 1⅓ cups flour ¼ tsp. salt 1 Tbs. sugar ½ cup butter, well chilled scant ⅓ cup ice water filling 2 lbs. firm pippin apples juice of 1 large lemon ½ cup sugar ½ to ⅓ cup apricot glaze (optional)

Directions: To make the crust, mix together the flour, salt, and 1 tablespoon of sugar, then cut in the butter with a pastry blender or two sharp knives until the mixture resembles coarse corn meal. Sprinkle the ice water over it and toss together quickly until the flour is evenly moistened and the dough is starting to hold together. Form the dough into a ball and chill it for 1 hour, then roll it out in a 12-inch circle and fit it into a 10½-inch false-bottom quiche tin or flan ring.* Trim off the excess, leaving a ¼-inch rim above the pan, and flute the rim with the blunt edge of a butter knife. Chill the shell for ½ hour. Line the shell with foil and fill it with dried beans or rice.• Bake in a preheated oven at 425 degrees for 8 minutes, then remove the beans and foil, prick the shell in several places with a fork, and put it back in the oven for 4 to 5 minutes, just until the bottom of the crust begins to color. Meanwhile, peel and core the apples and cut them in even, lengthwise slices, no thicker than ¼ inch at the outside. Put the apple slices in a bowl with the lemon juice and ½ cup of the sugar, toss lightly, and leave them there for 45 minutes. Drain the apples and reserve the liquid. The partially baked crust can be painted with apricot glaze before the apples are arranged on it. This is one more way to fight the soggy crust problem. Heat up the glaze and brush it on lightly with a pastry brush. Arrange the apple slices neatly in the crust by very closely overlapping them in concentric circles, starting at the outside edge. Use all the apples. Sprinkle the remaining sugar (about 3 tablespoons) evenly over the apples. Bake the tart for 30 to 35 minutes in a preheated oven at 375 degrees. The apples should just be starting to brown at the edges. While the tart is baking, boil the reserved liquid from the apples until it is reduced to a medium-thick, glazelike consistency. When the tart is done, brush the apples lightly with this glaze, or drizzle it over them. Serve the tart warm or cool, with or without the apricot glaze.

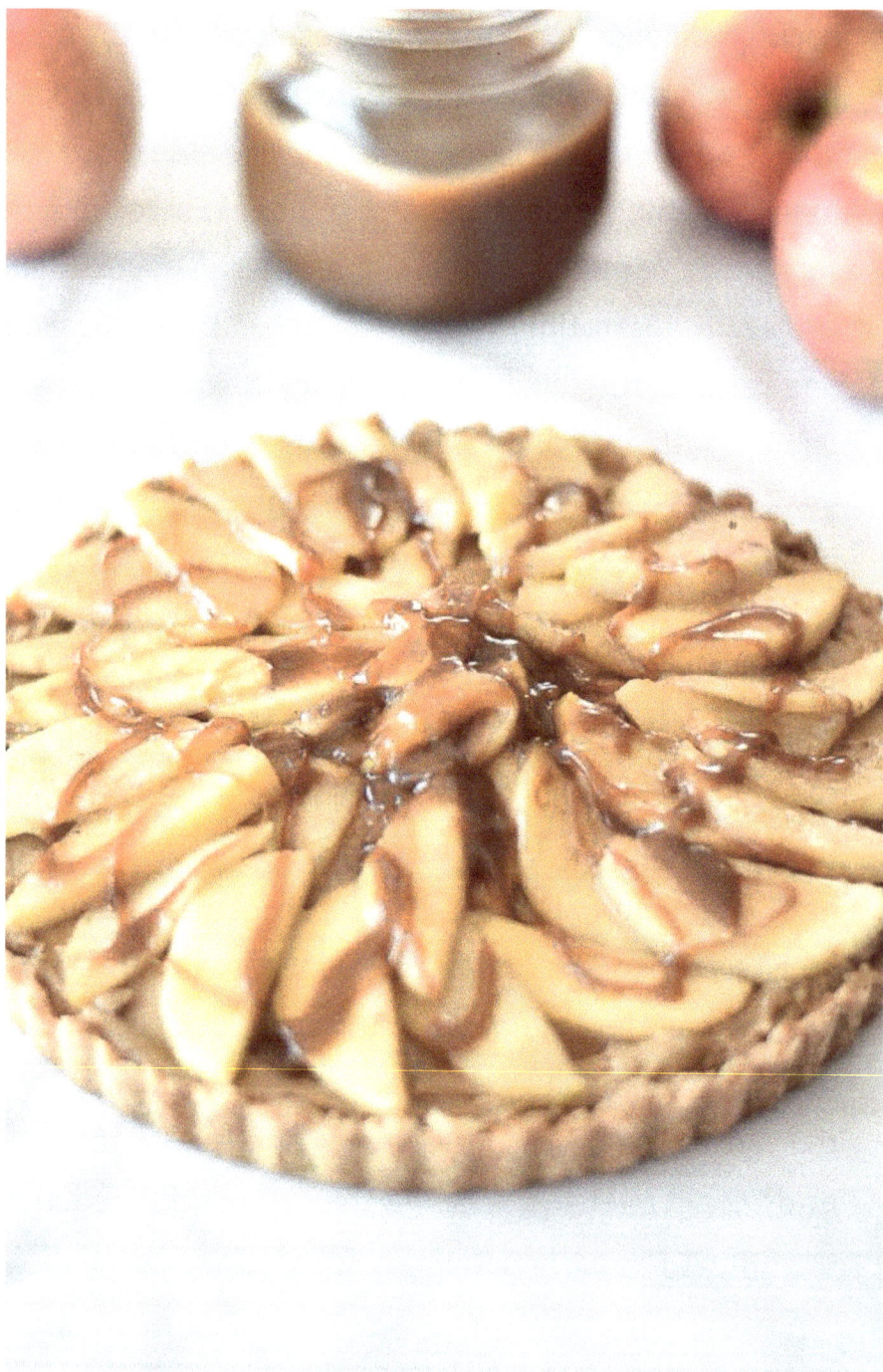

Lemon Torte

Preparation time: 5 minutesCooking time: 40 minutes
Servings: 2

Ingredients:

1¼ cups egg whites 2 cups confectioners' sugar 2 Tbs. cornstarch ¼ tsp. almond extract 1⅔ cups ground almonds (unblanched) Lemon Filling blanched almond halves

Directions:

Beat the egg whites with 1 cup of the confectioners' sugar until they hold soft peaks. Sift together the second cup of sugar and the cornstarch, add it to the egg whites along with the almond extract, and continue beating until the egg whites are stiff. Fold in the ground almonds. Butter and flour two 10-inch cake pans and divide the beaten egg white mixture between them, spreading it as flat and smooth as possible. Bake the layers in a preheated oven at 275 degrees for 1½ hours. They should be pale gold in color and shrinking away from the sides of the pan. Allow the layers to cool slightly in the pans, then carefully remove them and let them finish cooling on racks. Spread a little more than half the lemon filling on one layer and place the second layer on top of it. Spread the remaining filling over the top and sides of the top layer, leaving the sides of the bottom layer exposed. Decorate the torte very simply with a few blanched almond halves or just swirl the lemon topping evenly with a butter knife and leave it plain. Chill the torte for at least an hour.

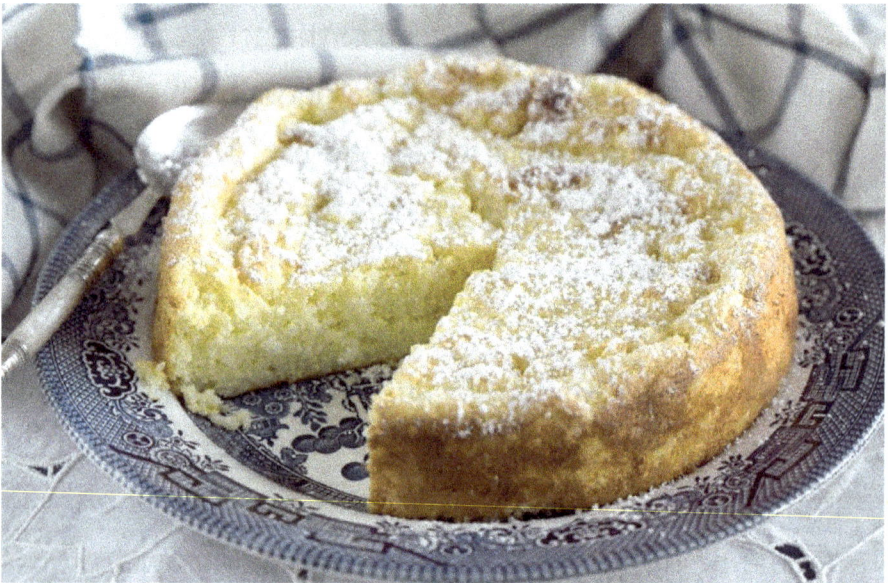

Nuts Balls

Preparation time: 10 minutes Cooking time: 20 minutes Servings: 12

Ingredients:

2 tablespoons flaxseed mixed with 3 tablespoons water 1 cup almonds, chopped 1 cup macadamia nuts, chopped ½ cup walnuts, chopped 1 cup coconut cream ¼ cup coconut, unsweetened and shredded ½ cup cashew cheese, grated Salt and black pepper to the taste 1 tablespoon Italian seasoning 2 tablespoons coconut oil, melted Cooking spray

Directions:

In a bowl, combine the flaxseed with the nuts, cream and the other ingredients except the cooking spray, whisk well and shape medium balls out of the mix. Arrange the balls on a baking sheet lined with parchment paper, grease with cooking spray and bake at 400 degrees F for 20 minutes. Arrange the balls on a platter and serve.

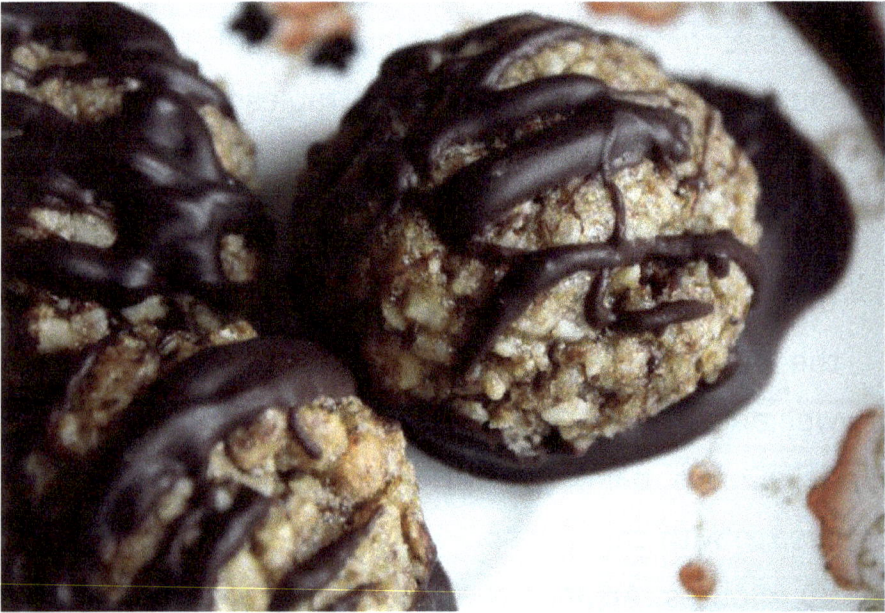

Kale & Avocado Smoothie

Preparation Time: 10 minutes Cooking Time: 0 minute Servings: 1

Ingredients:

1 ripe banana 1 cup kale 1 cup almond milk ¼ avocado 1 tbsp. chia seeds 2 tsp. honey 1 cup ice cubes

Direction:

Blend all the ingredients until smooth.

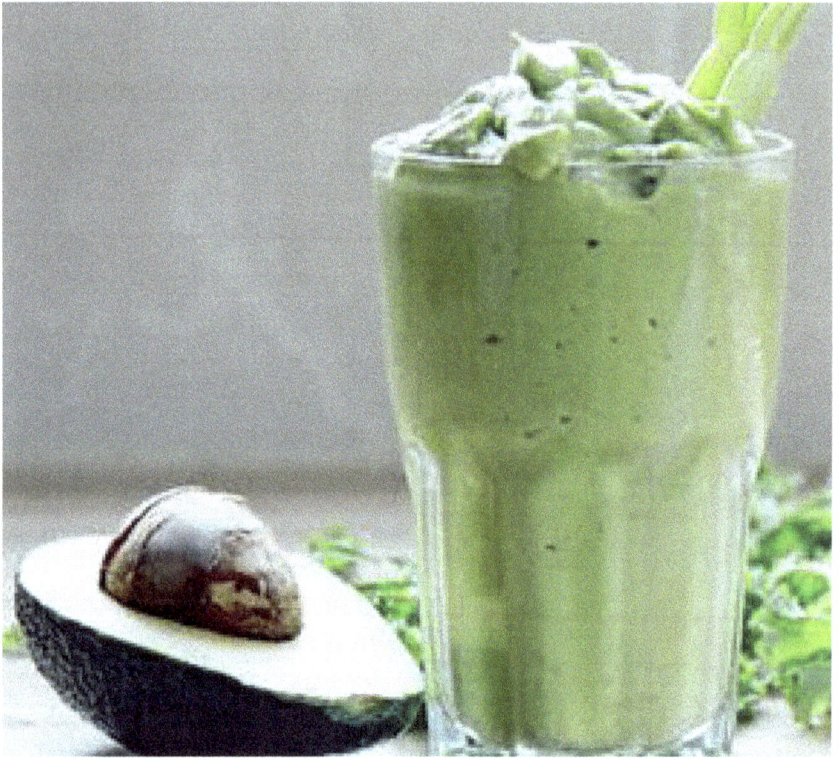

Orange & Carrot Juice

Preparation Time: 15 minutes Cooking Time: 0 minute Servings: 2

Ingredients:

1 tomato, sliced 1 orange, sliced into wedges 1 apple, sliced 4 carrots, sliced Ice cubes

Direction:

Follow the order of the ingredients list when processing these through the juice. Transfer the juice into glasses. Fill your glass with ice and serve.

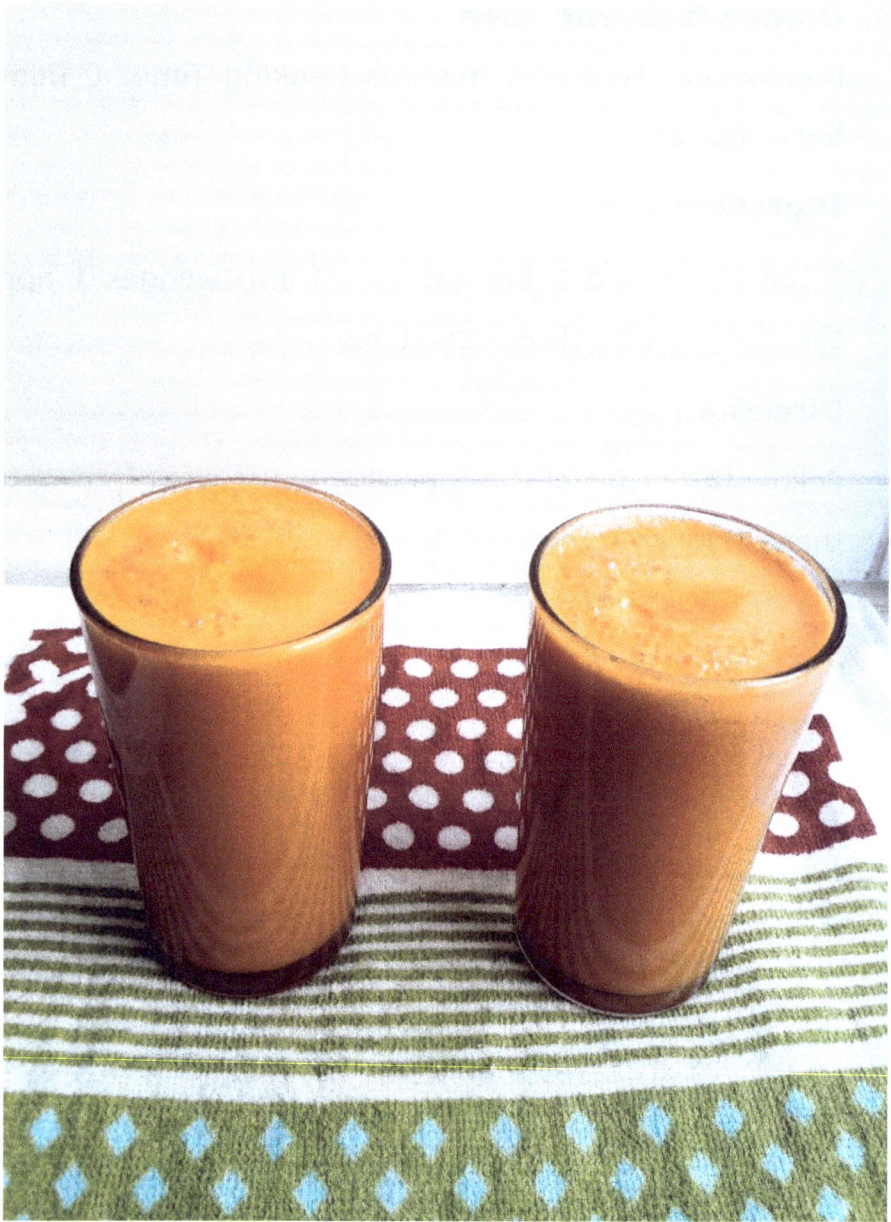

Sweet and Hot Nuts

Preparation time: 5 minutesCooking time: 4 hours; Servings: 12

Ingredients:

½ pound assorted nuts, raw 1/3 cup butter, melted 1 teaspoon cayenne pepper or to taste 1 tablespoon MCT oil or coconut oil What you'll need from the store cupboard: 1 packet stevia powder ¼ tsp salt

Directions

Place all ingredients in the crockpot. Give it a good stir to combine everything. Close the lid and cook on low for 4 hours.

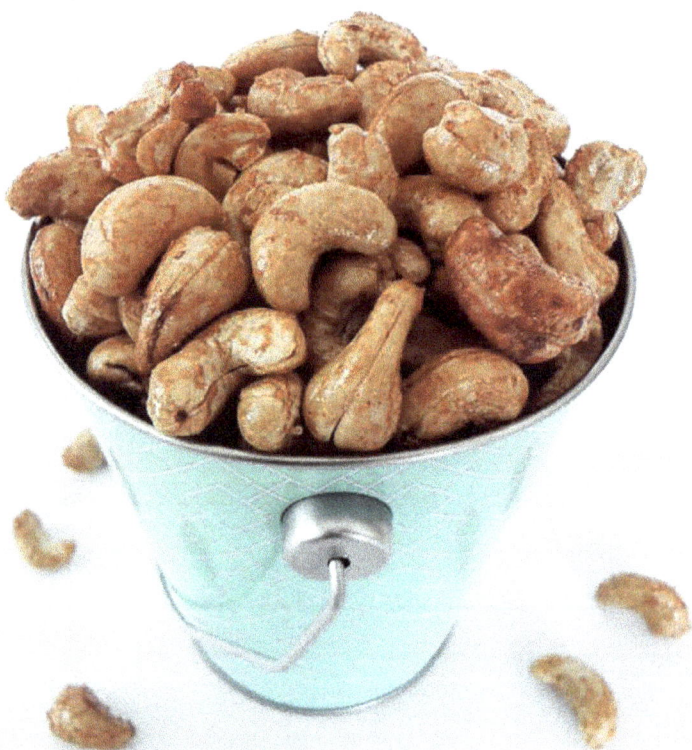

Sponge Cake

Preparation time: 5 minutesCooking time: 20 minutes
Servings: 4

Ingredients:

6 eggs, separated 1 cup sugar ¼ cup boiling water 1 Tbs. lemon juice ½ tsp. vanilla extract 1½ cups flour 1½ tsp. baking powder pinch of salt 4 Tbs. olive oil

Directions:

Beat the egg yolks until they are creamy and light, then gradually add the sugar a bit at a time, while you continue beating. Beat the yolks and sugar together until the mixture is pale colored and fluffy—another 10 minutes or so. Gradually add the boiling water, lemon juice, and vanilla and beat another few minutes. Sift together the flour and baking powder and fold it into the egg yolk mixture. Beat the egg whites with a pinch of salt until they hold firm peaks and fold them gently into the batter, using as few strokes as necessary. Pour olive oil butter over the batter, leaving out the milky sediment at the bottom of the pan. Again using as few strokes as necessary, in order not to deflate the egg whites, scoop in the butter. Spoon the batter into a buttered and floured 9-or 10-inch springform cake pan. Smooth the batter lightly in the pan.

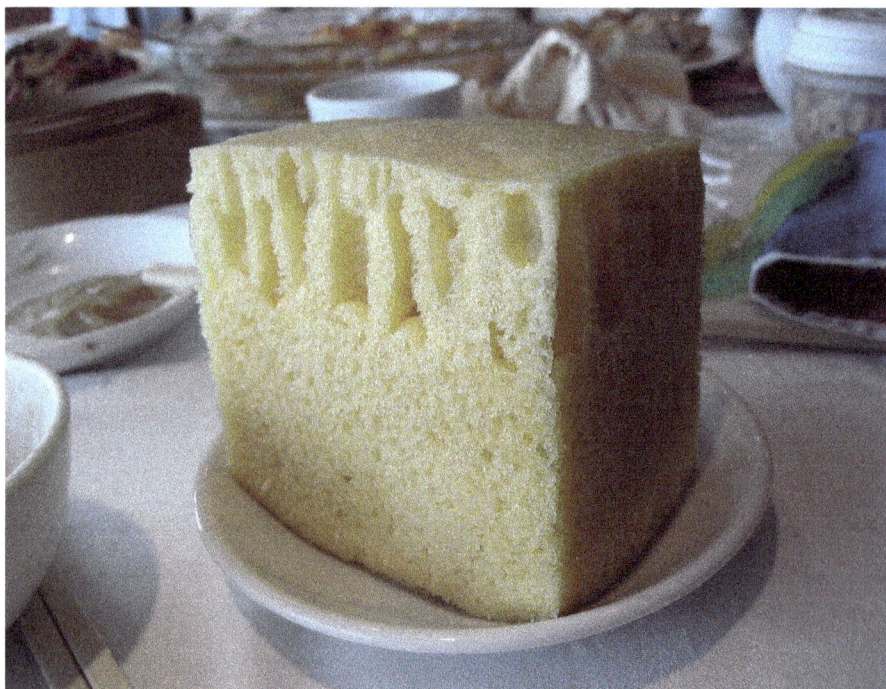

Mangoes with Cinnamon

Preparation time: 5 minutesCooking time: 20 minutes Servings: 4

Ingredients:

3 fresh mangoes 1 tsp. cinnamon

Directions: You will have two rounded sections of fruit and one flat section with the seed.. Slicing down to the skin but not through it, make cuts across the section about every half inch. Turn fruit 90 degrees and make another set of cuts. Hold the mango section in both hands. Using your fingers, push mango skin and turn inside out so the mango flesh will be removed from the cuts made and off the skin. Repeat with other side. Next, peel the middle section. Carefully slice the flesh from the seed. 2. Refrigerate mangoes overnight to chill thoroughly. Place in a dessert dish. Garnish with coconut and sprinkle lightly with cinnamon.

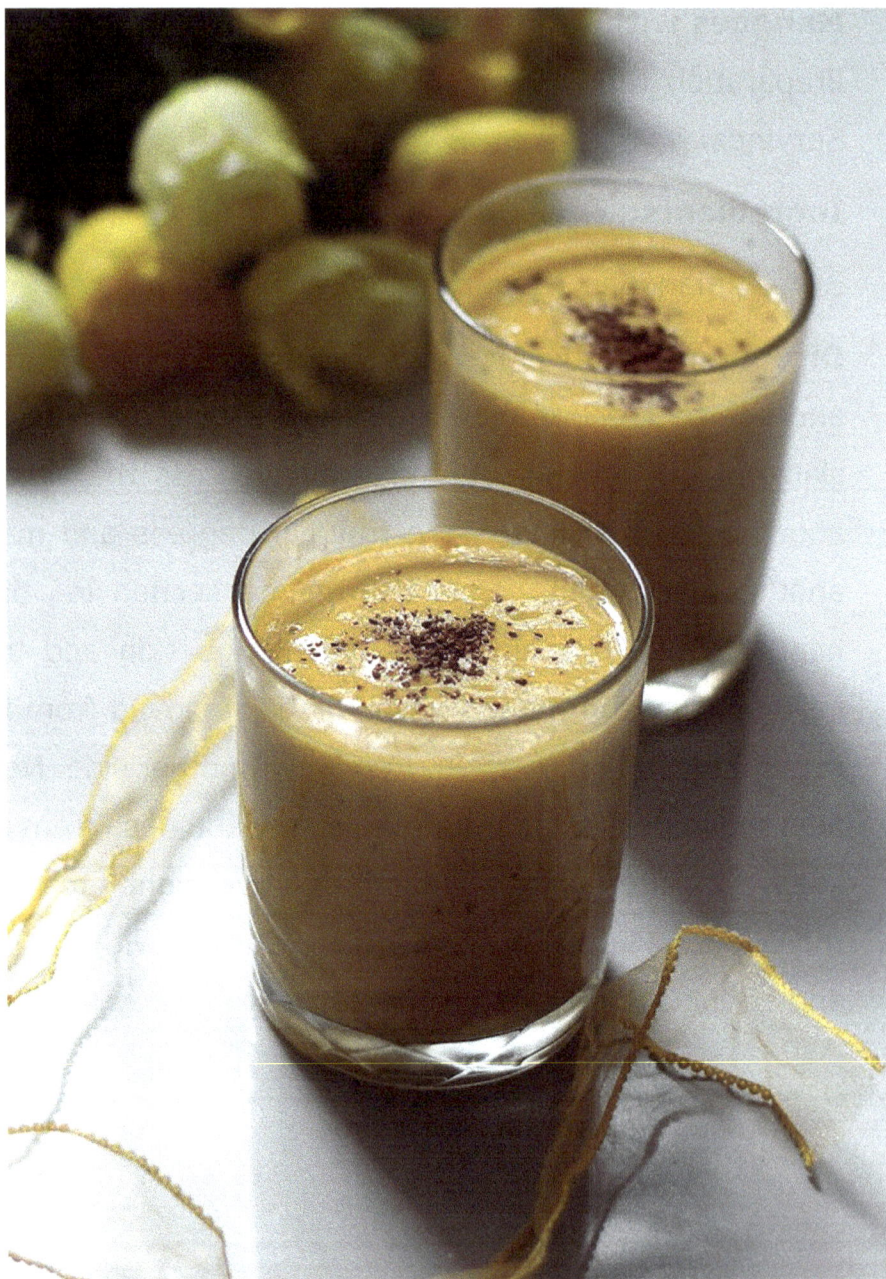

Apricot glaze

Preparation time: 5 minutesCooking time: 40 minutes Servings: 4

Ingredients

½ cup apricot preServings: or jam 1 Tbs. sugar

Directions: To make an apricot glaze, just rub the apricot preServings: or jam through a fine sieve, add the sugar, and boil for a few minutes. The mixture will be thick and sticky. Keep it warm over hot water until you need it, and while using it. If it gets too thick to handle, it can be thinned out with a few drops of water. *If you don't have a quiche pan or flan ring, a shallow 10-inch pie pan can be used, but I recommend getting a false-bottom quiche pan—they're inexpensive and very useful. †The dried beans or rice are used as a weight, to keep the crust from slipping down the sides and puffing up in the middle. Keep the beans or rice in a jar—they can be reused for this purpose indefinitely.

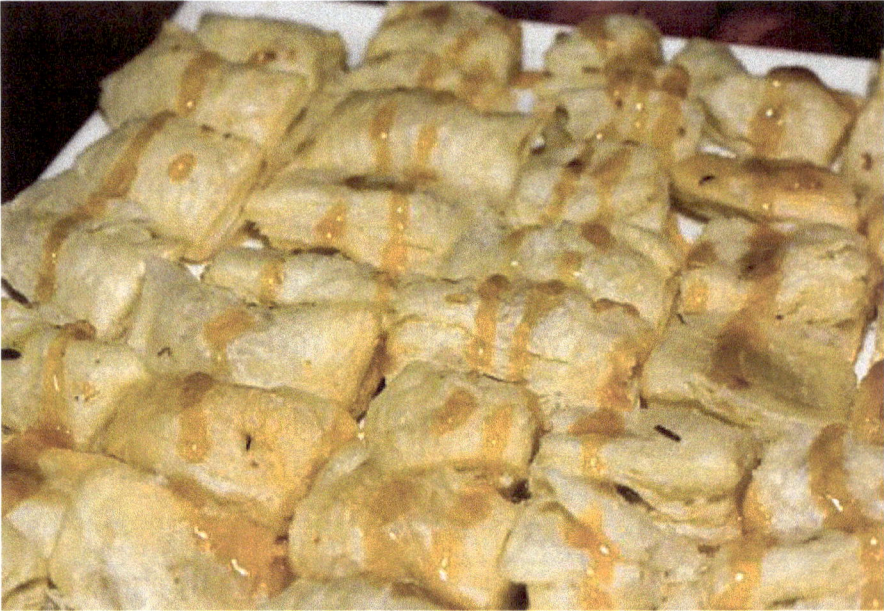

Acai and Banana Smoothie

Preparation time: 10 minutesCooking time: 0 minutes

Servings: 3

Ingredients:

1 cup of frozen acai ¼ cup of coconut milk 1 frozen banana ½ cup of frozen blueberries

Directions:

Put all the ingredients in the juicer or food processor and pulse until liquid. If needed, add some water to make it more liquid depending on the texture that you enjoy. Add a couple of ice cubes

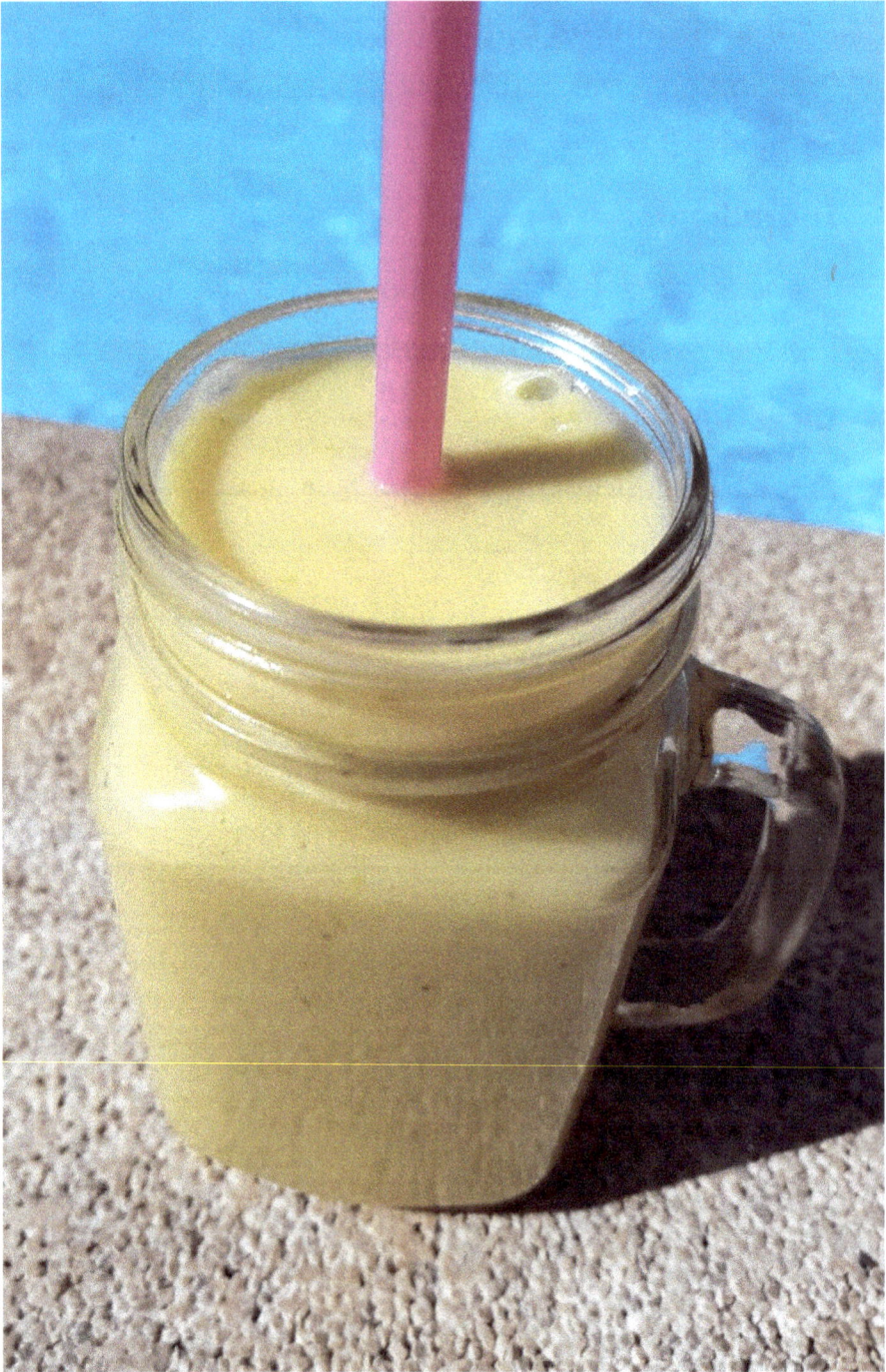

Berries Dip

Preparation time: 15 minutes Cooking time: 0 minutes Servings: 6

Ingredients:

1 cup blackberries 1 cup blueberries 1 cup coconut cream 1 teaspoon mint, dried 1 teaspoon stevia

Directions:

In a blender, combine the berries with the cream and the other ingredients, pulse well, divide into small bowls and keep in the fridge for 15 minutes before serving.

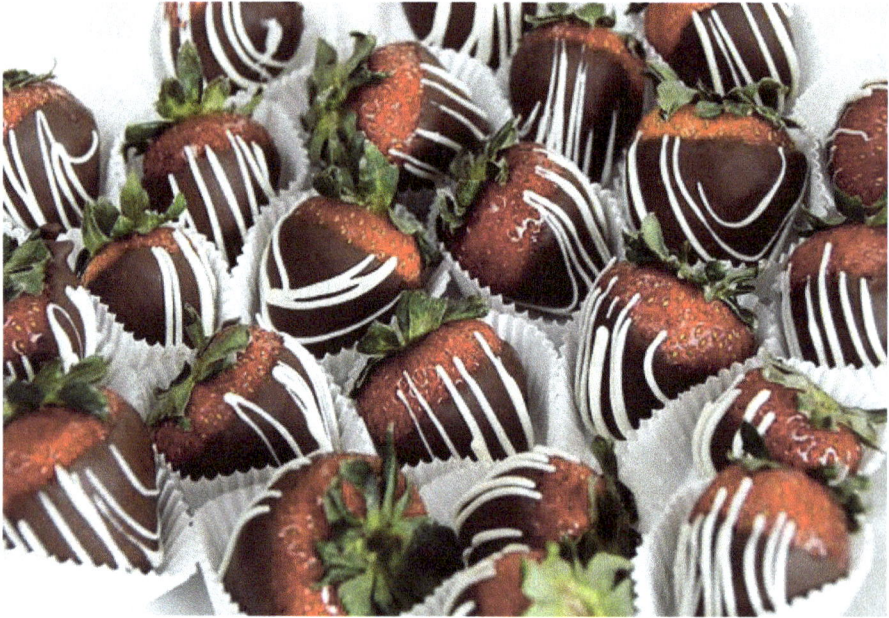

Blueberry and Greens Smoothie

Preparation time: 5 minutes Cooking time: 0 minutes Servings: 1

Ingredients:

¼ cup coconut milk 2 tbsps blueberries ½ cup arugula 1 tbsp hemp seeds What you'll need from the store cupboard: 2 packets Stevia, or as needed 1 ½ cups water 3 tbsps coconut oil

Directions

Add all ingredients in a blender. Blend until smooth and creamy. Serve and enjoy.

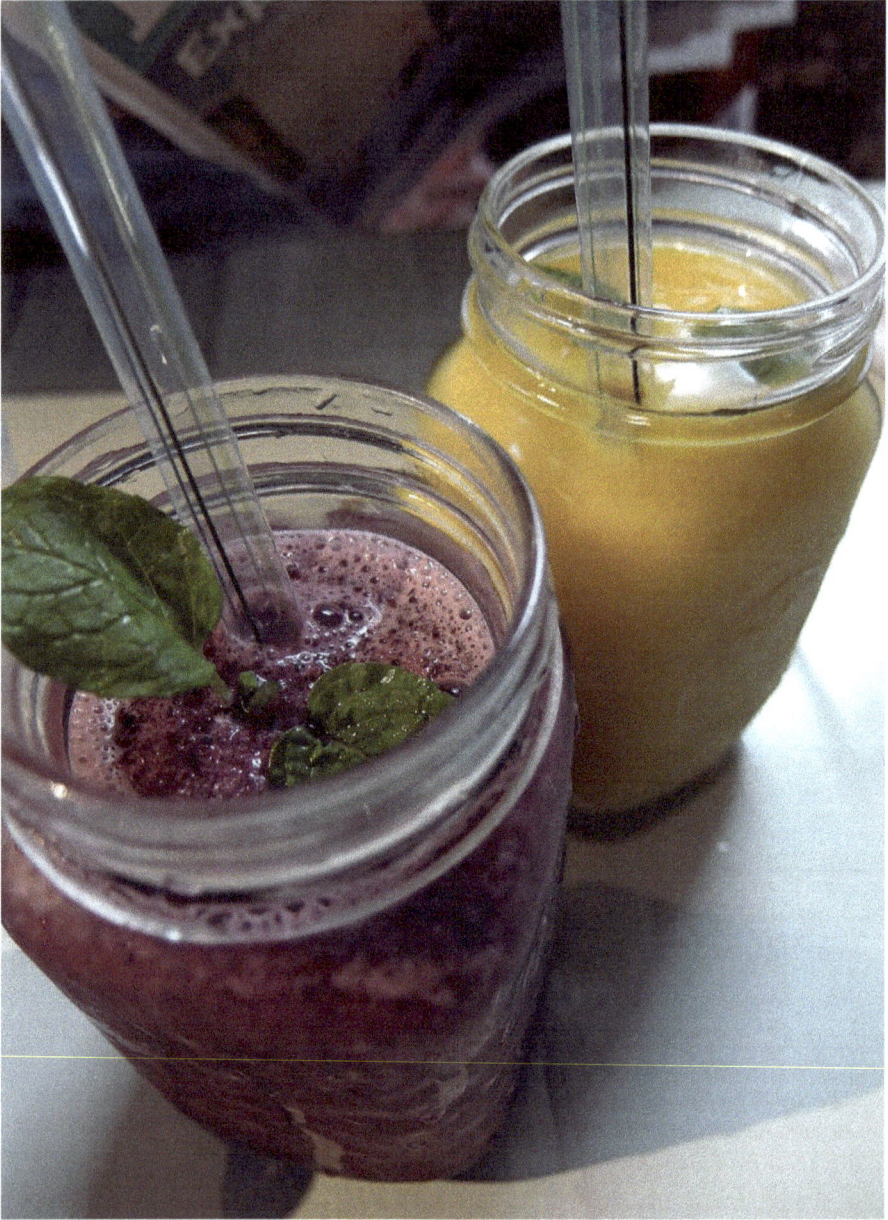

Boysenberry and Greens Shake

Preparation time: 5 minutes Cooking time: 0 minutes Servings: 1

Ingredients:

¼ cup coconut milk 2 tbsps Boysenberry 2 packets Stevia, or as needed ¼ cup Baby Kale salad mix 3 tbsps MCT oil What you'll need from the store cupboard: 1 ½ cups water

Directions

Add all ingredients in a blender. Blend until smooth and creamy. Serve and enjoy.

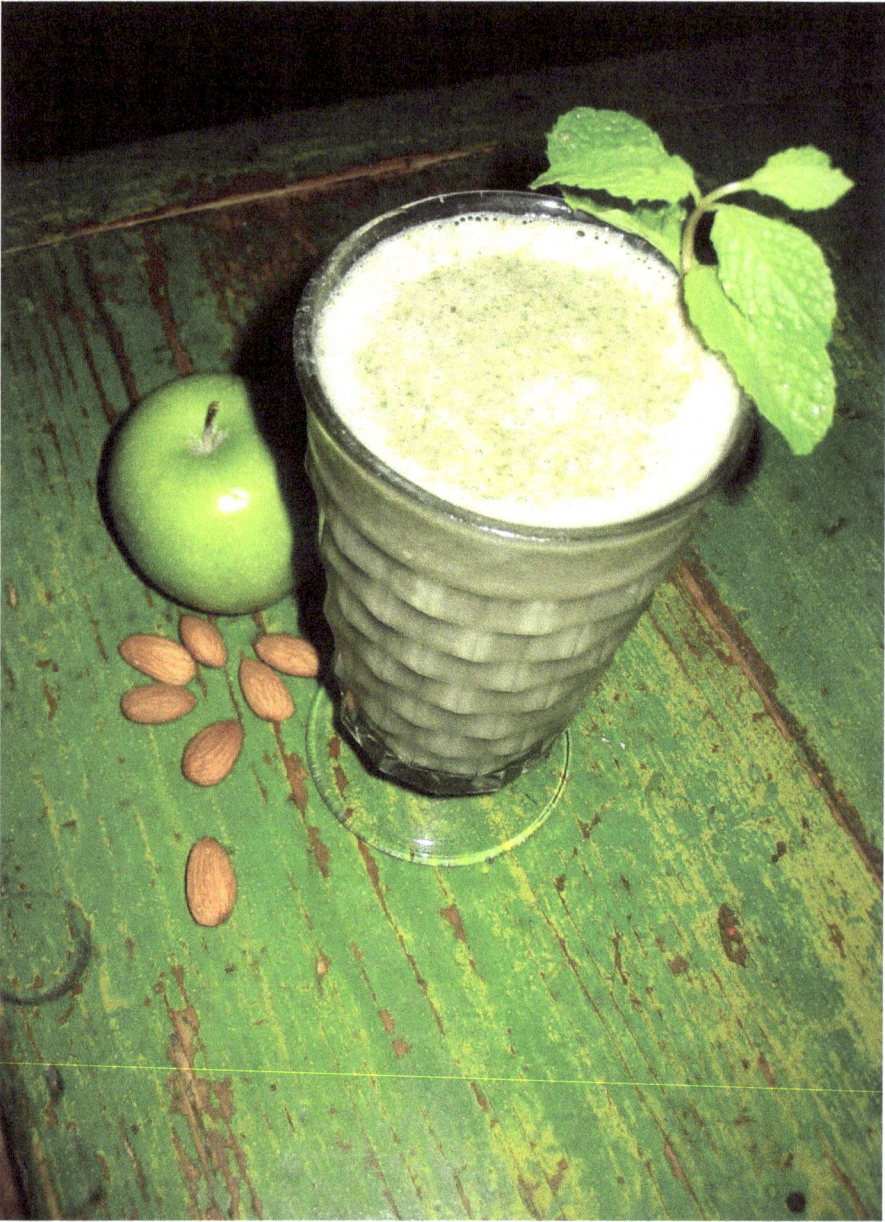